Fast Facts

D0528835

Fast Facts:
Minor Surgery

Second edition

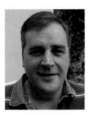

Christopher J Price MBBCh MRCGP DipMedEd
Associate Dean
Postgraduate Education for General Practice
Cardiff University
Cardiff, Wales, UK

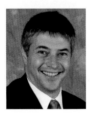

Rodney Sinclair MBBS MD FACD
Professor of Dermatology, University of Melbourne
Director of Dermatology Services,
St. Vincent's Hospital, Melbourne
Director of Research and Training
Skin and Cancer Foundation, Darlington/Westmead
New South Wales, Australia

Declaration of Independence
This book is as balanced and as practical as we can make it.
Ideas for improvement are always welcome: feedback@fastfacts.com

HEALTH PRESS

Fast Facts: Minor Surgery
First published 2001
Reprinted 2005, 2006
Second edition January 2008

Text © 2008 Christopher J Price, Rodney Sinclair
© 2008 in this edition Health Press Limited
Health Press Limited, Elizabeth House, Queen Street, Abingdon,
Oxford OX14 3LN, UK
Tel: +44 (0)1235 523233
Fax: +44 (0)1235 523238

Book orders can be placed by telephone or via the website.
For regional distributors or to order via the website, please go to:
www.fastfacts.com
For telephone orders, please call +44 (0)1752 202301 (UK and Europe),
1 800 247 6553 (USA, toll free), +1 419 281 1802 (Americas) or +61 (0)2 9351 6173
(Asia–Pacific).

Fast Facts is a trademark of Health Press Limited.

Figures in Chapter 3 are reproduced courtesy of the Department of Dermatology and
the Media Resources Centre, University Hospital of Wales, Cardiff, UK, and Medical
Illustration UK Ltd, Chelsea & Westminster Hospital, London, UK.

The publisher and the authors have made every effort to ensure the accuracy of this
book, but cannot accept responsibility for any errors or omissions.

For all drugs, please consult the product labeling approved in your country for
prescribing information.

A CIP record for this title is available from the British Library.

ISBN 978-1-903734-01-8

Price CJ (Christopher)
Fast Facts: Minor Surgery/
Christopher J Price, Rodney Sinclair

Medical illustrations by Dee McLean, London, UK.
Typesetting and page layout by Zed, Oxford, UK.
Printed by Fine Print (Services) Ltd, Oxford, UK.

Text printed with vegetable inks on biodegradable and
recyclable paper manufactured from sustainable forests.

Low
chlorine

Sustainable
forests

444 001
Low emissions
during production

Glossary of abbreviations

ABCD rule: a simple guide to the clinical features of melanoma (see page 36)

BCC: basal cell carcinoma

CNCH: chondrodermatitis nodularis chronica helicis

EFG: 'elevated', 'firm' and 'growing for more than 1 month'

EMLA®: eutectic mixture of local anesthetics

MM: malignant melanoma

PDT: photodynamic therapy

SCC: squamous cell carcinoma

Introduction

Dermatological surgery is practiced routinely in primary care, and most minor procedures are straightforward and require minimal time. Success depends on the practitioner's ability to recognize lesions, choose and plan appropriate treatment and perform surgical procedures.

This new edition of *Fast Facts: Minor Surgery* briefly describes the diagnosis of skin lesions, though the reader is encouraged to consult *Fast Facts: Skin Cancer* and other texts for more detail. The surgical techniques discussed and illustrated in this text are current best practice. These should be learned by supervised practice; this book is not an instruction manual for novices. All skin surgery causes scarring, and using the correct technique will only minimize this. The surgeon must always be confident that the procedure is necessary and that the likely degree of scarring is appropriate for the type of lesion, particularly when treating benign skin conditions.

A patient may request removal of a benign lesion purely to improve their cosmetic appearance. Before such surgery is contemplated, the surgeon should be satisfied that the outcome will improve the appearance of the patient. Furthermore, the patient must be made aware that the lesion is benign and that there is potential for scarring and complications.

During surgery, the patient's skin, which is the first line of defense against invading pathogens, will be breached, making him or her more vulnerable to cross-infection. It is therefore important that the surgeon and any assistants are free from bacterial or viral infection to reduce this risk. Conversely, staff are potentially at risk of infection from the patient, and every effort should be made to avoid needle-stick injury and to minimize handling of infected tissue. Finally, any excised specimens (including lesions believed to be benign) should be sent for pathological examination, and the report read, recorded and acted on by the surgeon.

This second edition of *Fast Facts: Minor Surgery* provides an overview of the good practice and operative set-up required for dermatological surgery, the skin lesions commonly encountered in primary care and the various techniques and procedures involved in their treatment. It is hoped that the information presented will benefit you, your colleagues and your patients.

The minimum requirements for safe practice-based surgery are discussed in this chapter. It is vital that any operative intervention is performed in a facility set up for the purpose, with proper regard to sterile procedure. Access to equipment to deal with potential complications should be a prerequisite; training and confidence to use these facilities will ensure patient (and operator) safety.

Operating facilities

Room. The shape and size of the operating room is usually dictated by available space. However, space around the couch must be sufficient for access with an operating trolley and there should be access at the head for airway protection should the patient faint. Resuscitation equipment must be easily accessible in the same room. A clean sink for hand-washing and a dedicated 'dirty area' for used instruments and dirty swabs must also be provided. Adequate work surfaces and storage facilities should also be available.

Lighting. The operating room should have bright background lighting to ensure operator and assistant safety. If the operating field is well lit but the remainder of the room is dim, used instruments or sharps on the operating trolley may be overlooked, resulting in needle-stick injury. It is also safer in the event of a patient requiring resuscitation.

The surgical light should be mounted on a flexible arm to allow variation in focus. This can be achieved conveniently with a ceiling-mounted lamp. Floor-based lamps are adequate but leave trailing wires that can be dangerous. Also, the surgical light should not emit too much heat as this may cause the patient or surgeon discomfort during long procedures and can lead to drying of surgically exposed tissues. Many 'cold' lights are available.

Couch. The type of couch required for the operating room will depend on the surgeon's preference and the type of operations performed. If long complex operations are undertaken, a good-quality couch, with the facilities for height adjustment and tilting the patient into a head-down position, together with a multiposition backrest, is essential. If the couch is used for small procedures only, such as curettage and cautery, then a static one is adequate.

Resuscitation equipment. Minor surgery inevitably involves some blood loss and the use of local anesthetic. Although it is unlikely that patients will be hemodynamically compromised, some may faint from the psychological effect of seeing their own blood. Also, local anesthesia carries a small risk of syncope, allergy or, much less frequently, anaphylaxis, so a patient may need cardiac and/or respiratory support. Resuscitation facilities should always be close at hand in the same room in case of either a vasovagal or anaphylactic attack.

Table 1.1 shows the minimum requirements and optional extras for resuscitation equipment. The operator and assistant should be fully trained to use the equipment, which must also be regularly inspected and maintained. It is a good idea to keep a laminated sheet showing drug doses printed in large typeface with the equipment; in an emergency, this is one thing less to worry about.

Cautery. Simple heat cautery units are inexpensive and are sufficient for all but the most complex skin surgery. If more complex surgery is undertaken, or if the practice has a large turnover of operations, then an electrocautery unit may be a viable alternative. An electrocautery unit can be used in deep wounds and achieves hemostasis with less tissue damage. These units are expensive and are not necessary for superficial surgery or minor excisions in which bleeding can be controlled by pressure or tying off blood vessels.

Chemical agents for hemostasis include aluminum hydrochloride, trichloroacetic acid, phenol and silver nitrate (Table 1.2). These agents act either by precipitating proteins, thus triggering coagulation pathways, or by simple tissue destruction. Chemical cautery is used mainly for superficial wounds following shave excision or curettage.

TABLE 1.1
Equipment and drugs for resuscitation

Essential
- Airways in various sizes
- Artificial ventilation (ambu-bag)
- Oxygen
- Intravenous cannulas
- Epinephrine (adrenaline) 1:1000
- Diazepam, 5 mg injectable
- Chlorpheniramine, 10 mg injectable
- Needles and syringes

Optional extras
- Electrocardiogram
- Defibrillation unit
- Intravenous fluids
- Intubation equipment
- Injectable steroid (e.g. hydrocortisone, 100 mg)

Support staff

It is advisable always to operate with an assistant who is familiar with:
- resuscitation equipment and techniques
- sterile procedures
- the range of instruments required for the operation
- stock items, such as drugs, sutures and dressings.

Usually, the assistant will not need to scrub for minor procedures but should know how to do so if more complex procedures are undertaken or an extra pair of hands is required, for example if a patient bleeds excessively. The ideal assistant should be calm, able to reassure the patient and capable of observing them at all times for signs of distress or adverse reaction.

TABLE 1.2

Chemical agents used in cautery

Agent	Advantages	Disadvantages
Aluminum hydrochloride (20–50%)	• Lack of tissue necrosis • No tattooing	• Irritant to eyes
Trichloroacetic acid (30–50%)	• Strongly hemostatic	• May damage surrounding epithelium
Phenol (50–100%)	• Strongly hemostatic	• May damage surrounding epithelium
Silver nitrate (20–50%)	• Germicidal	• Slow acting • Variable success • Potential to tattoo

Spills and contamination

Caustic substances. Written protocols should exist in case of spillage of caustic materials within the operating room. Such materials should be stored in a locked cupboard.

Dirty or infected material and sharps should be disposed of away from the clean operating area. Swabs contaminated with body fluids should be wrapped and stored for disposal in an area not accessible to patients. Sharps should be placed directly into disposal boxes for incineration – again, these items should not be accessible to the public. It is the surgeon's personal responsibility to ensure that sharps are disposed of appropriately; it may therefore be advisable for surgeons to deposit needles and blades directly into the sharps box themselves. At the very least, sharps should be accounted for and piled on a corner of the operating trolley for disposal by the assistant. Used instruments should be scrubbed clean of small pieces of tissue and stored for re-sterilization in a safe area away from the clean environment.

Blood spills onto the operating floor should be scrubbed with disinfectant immediately after the procedure. The operating couch and all surgical workbenches should be wiped down between operations. The theatre should be professionally cleaned on a regular basis, the frequency of which will depend on the range and number of procedures performed and the potential for contamination. Staff should refer to local infection control policies.

Prevention of infection

The operating room for minor skin surgery needs to be clinically clean but not necessarily sterile. Minimizing risk from potential sources of infection should be a matter of routine and vigilance (Table 1.3).

TABLE 1.3

Prevention of wound infection

Potential source of infection	Preventative measures
Operator and assistant	• Ensure hand-washing and correct 'gloving-up' technique (see Figure 1.3, page 15) • Free from skin infection or nasal contamination • Good sterile field technique • Avoid glove puncture; immediately change glove and needle in the event of a needle-stick injury
Patient	• Prepare skin • Drape with sterile towels • Administer peri- or postoperative antibiotics (if lesion is infected or dirty) • Postoperative wound dressing and advice
Environment	• A clinically clean operating room • Storage of dirty material for disposal away from the clean environment • Good ventilation • All surfaces (floor, walls, ceiling, worktops) in good repair

CONTINUED

TABLE 1.3 (CONTINUED)

Potential source of infection	Preventative measures
Equipment	• Clean instruments of tissue debris before correct sterilization • Sterilize cautery unit between patients • Sterile dressings and swabs • Sterile packs
Pre-operatively	• The patient should avoid shaving hairy areas for at least 24 hours before the procedure • Give antibiotics when required • Remove the crust from infected tumors 48 hours before the procedure and dress with iodine • Stop acetylsalicylic acid (aspirin), if possible, 7–14 days before the procedure
Operative technique	• Minimize tissue damage and blood in wound • Good hemostatic techniques, allowing drainage of infected wounds (e.g. abscesses) • Remove all non-viable tissue from abscesses and allow them to granulate
Postoperatively	• Use semi-occlusive dressing for 48 hours • Keep wounds dry for at least 48 hours • Avoid excessive movement of wound

The sterile field. To minimize the risk of wound infection, it is important to establish and maintain a sterile operating field, which includes:

• the area of the patient being operated on
• the surrounding sterile drapes
• the surgeon's (and assistant's) gloved hands
• the top of the instrument trolley covered with a sterile drape
• any swabs used
• instruments and sutures on the trolley (Figure 1.1).

The sterile field should be established in stages (Figure 1.2). The operating trolley should have a steel or glass surface that can be cleaned easily with disinfectant.

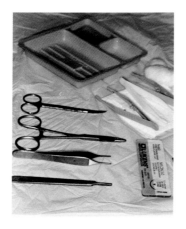
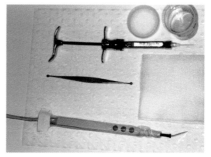

Figure 1.1 Surgical instruments should be set up on a trolley on a sterile drape.

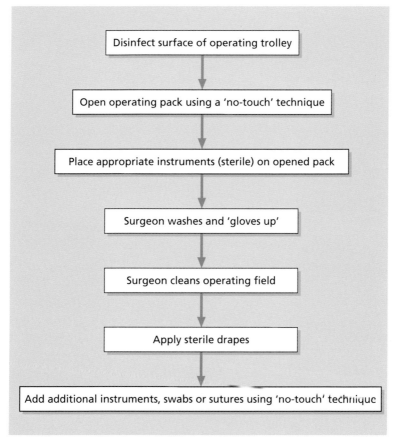

Disinfect surface of operating trolley

↓

Open operating pack using a 'no-touch' technique

↓

Place appropriate instruments (sterile) on opened pack

↓

Surgeon washes and 'gloves up'

↓

Surgeon cleans operating field

↓

Apply sterile drapes

↓

Add additional instruments, swabs or sutures using 'no-touch' technique

Figure 1.2 Setting up a sterile operating field.

13

A sterile operating pack containing swabs and towels should be opened using a 'no-touch' technique. If the instruments are not included, then correctly sterilized instruments should be placed on the pack, again without contaminating either the instruments or operating pack.

The surgeon washes, 'gloves up' (this is best taught practically by someone experienced in the technique; Figure 1.3) and may now use the sterile field created on the top of the trolley.

Skin-preparation fluid is used to clean the operative area and surrounding skin on the patient. The choice of skin preparation is an individual one, as none is ideal. Alcohol-based solutions should not be used with cautery or electrocautery (diathermy) because of the fire risk. The most commonly used solutions are povidone-iodine and aqueous chlorhexidine.

The operating area should be draped with sterilized linen or water-resistant paper towels. The surgeon should take care not to touch anything outside the areas prepared, and the assistant (unless scrubbed) should not touch areas within the sterile field.

Sutures, extra swabs and instruments should be deposited onto the sterile field using a 'no-touch' technique. If the sterile field is accidentally contaminated, it should be re-established to the highest possible standard.

Other precautions. Establishment of a sterile field and constant vigilance minimize potential infection of the patient. However, the risk of cross-infection from the patient to the surgeon or assistant should also be considered.

Bloodborne viral infections, such as hepatitis B and HIV, are the main threat but superficial skin infections may be transmitted if the surgeon's skin is compromised. Active immunization against hepatitis B should be mandatory for both surgeon and assistant, and procedures to prevent needle-stick injury should be in place. A written protocol of action should be available in case of needle-stick injury. The protocol will depend on local guidelines, and may be available from a local microbiology department.

It is also advisable for surgeons to wear protective glasses to prevent blood splashing into their eyes during the operation.

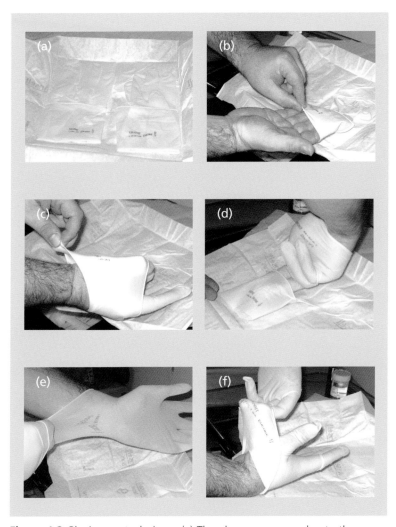

Figure 1.3 Gloving-up technique. (a) The gloves are opened onto the sterile pack using a no-touch technique. (b) The cuffs of the gloves are folded back on themselves – it is important that the surgeon's skin touches only the inside of the glove. Here the inside of the right glove is held by the surgeon's left hand. (c) The right glove is pulled on, leaving the cuff folded back over the thumb. (d) The left glove is held with the (sterile-gloved) right hand. (e) The left glove is pulled on and the cuff is turned back correctly. (f) The right cuff is turned back correctly. The gloves may need minor adjustments on the fingers – the gloved hands are now sterile.

15

Sterilization of instruments. Any instruments that are to be reused must be sterilized. This can be achieved either on the premises using a bench-top autoclave or by arrangement with a local sterile supplies department. Boiling does not render instruments completely sterile and the practice is no longer considered safe. Sterilization removes all pathogens including viruses, fungi, bacteria and bacterial spores.

The first stage of sterilization is physical cleaning of used instruments to remove pieces of tissue, otherwise the sterilization process may be hindered. Bench-top autoclaves must be operated in line with the manufacturer's instructions and should be serviced and tested regularly; a logbook of their service history and test results should be kept. As a minimum requirement, sterilization procedures and standards should adhere to local regulations.

Surgical instruments

Surgical instruments have evolved and developed over many years. Most are eponymously named and have individual features that different surgeons grow accustomed to. Choice of instruments for skin surgery depends on personal preference; however, sufficient instruments to perform the planned procedure and deal with any problems that arise must be available. For example, artery forceps are essential in case of excessive bleeding.

Scalpel handle (No. 3) and blade (No. 15). The No. 15 blade is ideal for most skin surgery (Figure 1.4). It has a small, easily controlled cutting surface, shaped to facilitate straight and sure incisions that start and finish at 90° to the skin surface. Larger blades tend to be more clumsy and so are not advisable for delicate skin work. Disposable scalpels with plastic handles are available as an alternative.

Tissue forceps (Figure 1.5) should be used to grip the excision specimen and to offer up the edge of the wound for suture insertion. It is not good practice to use non-gripping (dressing) forceps, as the pressure applied may crush the wound edges. It is preferable to potentially puncture, rather than crush, the wound as crushing will impede healing.

A skin hook (Figure 1.6) may be preferred to tissue forceps for work on wound edges. If manipulated with care and dexterity, a skin hook will cause less tissue damage and crushing.

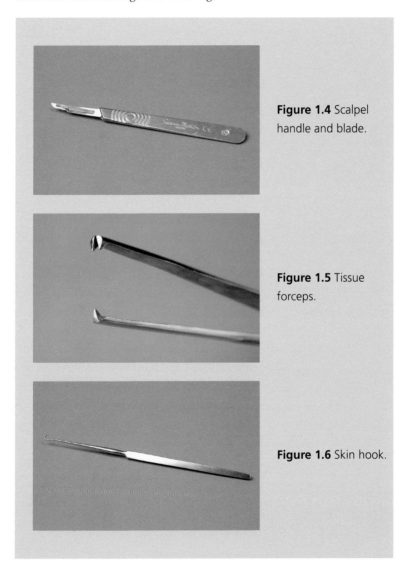

Figure 1.4 Scalpel handle and blade.

Figure 1.5 Tissue forceps.

Figure 1.6 Skin hook.

Scissors are used to perform a number of tasks in skin surgery, including cutting tissue, undermining, and cutting sutures following placement. The blades may be straight or curved, and are available with sharp or rounded tips (Figure 1.7). Straight sharp-tipped Iris scissors are useful for cutting tissue.

Most surgeons prefer to use rounded-tipped curved scissors for tissue dissection and undermining, as there is more control over positioning of the blade and less chance of puncturing overlying skin with the rounded ends. Choice of scissors depends on personal preference, but the golden rules are that they should be very sharp and that the blades should oppose smoothly to enable cutting of tissue without crushing.

Separate scissors should be used for cutting sutures, as this may quickly blunt surgical scissors.

Needle holders (Figure 1.8). Many different types are available, but for skin surgery the holder needs to be short, with small jaws that are either very finely serrated or non-serrated. Fine suture material can be damaged by serrations and the small jaws avoid flattening out the curve in fine needles. The Webster needle holder with smooth jaws is a logical first choice.

Artery forceps (hemostats) (Figure 1.9) are used to clamp the larger veins and arterioles that are inevitably cut during surgery. They should be available during all incisional surgery performed without sophisticated hemostatic electrocautery equipment. Artery forceps are available with straight or curved blades and have serrated surfaces; the Halsted mosquito is commonly used. A minimum of six artery forceps must be available to be added to the instrument trolley if required during the procedure.

Curettes are invaluable instruments for the skin surgeon. Semi-sharp reusable curettes, such as the Volkmann curette, are useful for softer, more friable lesions. The disposable sharp curette has a circular loop, one edge of which is a surgical blade while the opposite edge may be used for 'blunt' curettage. Both types are available in a number of sizes (Figure 1.10).

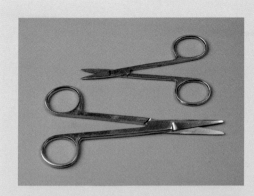

Figure 1.7 Sharp-tipped (top) and rounded-tipped (bottom) surgical scissors.

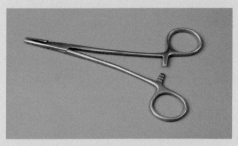

Figure 1.8 Needle holder.

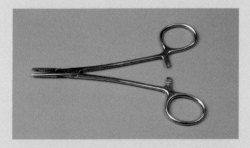

Figure 1.9 Artery forceps.

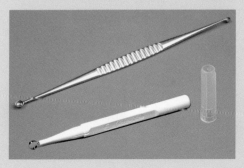

Figure 1.10 Curettes: Volkmann (top) and disposable (bottom).

Suture material

Choice of suture material affects the final appearance of the wound.
Sutures are classified as either 'absorbable' if the material is absorbed by
the body or 'non-absorbable' if it is not. Absorbable sutures are used in
subcutaneous tissue to reduce skin tension at the surface and to give the
wound strength while the scar matures. Non-absorbable sutures are
usually used to approximate the skin surface and are removed within
7–14 days. Many different types of suture are commercially available,
and the surgeon's preference will determine the type used (Tables 1.4
and 1.5).

In skin surgery, sutures are usually mounted on a reverse-cutting
curved needle. The cutting tip of the needle is triangular in outline. The
apex of the triangle points away from the wound, helping to minimize

TABLE 1.4

Non-absorbable sutures

Suture	Advantages	Disadvantages	Uses
Silk	• Easy to tie • Handles well with no memory • Soft	• Bioactive • May be colonized by microorganisms	In areas where cosmetic appearance is less important
Ethilon®	• Monofilament • Relatively inert • Has the least memory of the synthetic monofilament sutures	• Black color may be difficult to identify in hair (blue-dyed Ethilon® is available)	All superficial skin suturing
Prolene®	• Monofilament • Relatively inert • Bright blue; easily identified in the hair	• Memory is greatest of all monofilament sutures	All superficial skin suturing, particularly useful in hair
Novafil®	• Monofilament • Relatively inert • High degree of elasticity; expands and contracts slightly with the wound tissues	• Intermediate memory	All superficial skin suturing

any tendency of the suture to cut into the tissue surrounding the wound. Sutures are sized according to the approximate cross-section of the material. The higher the number in front of the '0', the thinner the material; for example, 4-0 is thicker than 6-0.

Suture material may attempt to revert to its original configuration; if this occurs it is said to have 'memory'. This is not a desirable characteristic as knots may untie; this is a particular problem with synthetic monofilament sutures.

Absorbable sutures vary in composition and this variation defines their respective properties. Polymerized materials that are dissolved by the body with a much-reduced inflammatory response, such as polyglycolic acid (Dexon®), polyglactin (Vicryl®) and polydioxanone (PDS®), have superseded catgut and are now commonly used.

TABLE 1.5

Absorbable sutures

Suture	Advantages	Disadvantages	Uses
Dexon®	• Less inflammatory response than with catgut • Excellent knot security	• Intermediate longevity within wound	Buried sutures in all areas
Vicryl®	• Less inflammatory response than with catgut • Excellent knot security • More pliable and retains tensile strength longer than Dexon®		Buried sutures in all areas
PDS®	• Less inflammatory response than with catgut • Retains tensile strength longer than Vicryl®	• Has less pliability and more memory • Knots may be less secure	Excellent for wounds under greatest tension or in areas where movement occurs, e.g. upper trunk

Key points – operative set-up and equipment

- Proper regard to sterile procedure is an essential requirement of any operative set-up.
- Resuscitation equipment must be regularly inspected and maintained, and easily accessible during the procedure.
- The ideal assistant should be calm, reassuring and vigilant.
- Written protocols should exist in case of spillage of caustic materials.
- Dirty and infected materials and sharps must be inaccessible to patients.
- Reusable instruments must be sterilized; boiling does not render instruments sterile.
- Skin marking before administration of anesthetic is advisable to ensure accurate, straight and sure incisions.
- Choice of suture material affects the final appearance of the wound.

Appropriate use of local anesthesia is vital for safe surgical practice and for patient comfort. Common methods of achieving anesthesia before skin surgery include:
- topical application
- local tissue infiltration
- nerve block.

Topical application

Anesthetic agents have been applied topically for many years. They range from cold sprays and ice, to topical lidocaine in jellies and sprays, and more recently, EMLA® cream (eutectic mixture of local anesthetics). EMLA® cream is applied as a thick layer under an occlusive dressing at least 1 hour before surgery (longer for thicker skin). Although the duration and effectiveness of the anesthesia vary, EMLA® provides an alternative route of anesthesia for superficial skin surgery and is useful in nervous patients and children. EMLA® cream may also be used before local tissue infiltration to lessen the discomfort of the injection.

Local tissue infiltration

This involves injection of anesthetic either into the deep dermis or just deep to the dermis in the subcutaneous fat layer. Various injectable anesthetics are available with different properties, speed of onset and duration of action. The most commonly used is lidocaine, which has a rapid onset and a duration of action of 1–1.5 hours. It is available as plain lidocaine (0.5–2%) or pre-mixed with epinephrine (adrenaline) in 1:80 000–1:200 000 solutions. Addition of epinephrine retards the onset of anesthesia and increases its duration of action by reducing reabsorption. This effect also allows larger volumes of anesthetic to be used safely.

A variation on local infiltration is the field block, in which the operating field is rendered anesthetic by infiltrating a ring of anesthesia around it (Figure 2.1). This has the benefit of not distorting skin within the area being operated on.

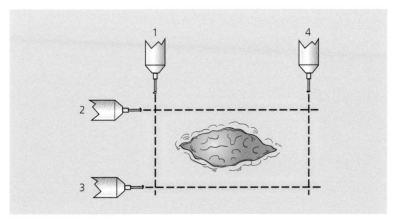

Figure 2.1 A field block. Four injection points are used around the lesion. The blue shaded area represents the extent of infiltration of anesthetic.

Nerve block

A nerve block renders an area anesthetic by blocking the sensory nerve that supplies it. The techniques and regional sites of the many possible nerve blocks are best learned by practical experience. The *Atlas of Cutaneous Surgery* is a useful source of reference (see Further reading, page 114).

The most commonly used nerve block is the digital ring block, which involves infiltrating anesthetic without epinephrine around the digital nerve at the level of the web space. For a great toe, 1–2 mL of lidocaine (1%) is required either side of the proximal phalanx and a further 0.5 mL is injected over the dorsal aspect because a branch of the digital nerve may pass over the proximal phalanx at this point. The main complication of a ring block is puncturing the digital artery. This is of little importance unless the circulation was compromised previously, for example in diabetes or peripheral vascular disease.

Adverse effects

Lidocaine is well tolerated and relatively non-toxic when used correctly. It has a maximum safe dose in local anesthesia of 200 mg (40 mL of 0.5% solution, 20 mL of 1% solution or 10 mL of 2% solution). Most minor procedures require 1–2 mL of anesthetic and even a ring block requires a maximum of 3–5 mL. Addition of epinephrine extends the duration of action of the anesthetic and creates a relatively bloodless operating field by inducing vasoconstriction. In areas supplied by end arteries, such as digits or the penis, the risk of inducing prolonged ischemia distal to the injection site makes the combined preparation unsuitable for use; however, on the nose and ears, the rich supply of blood means that epinephrine is an asset not a risk.

Key points – local anesthesia

- Common methods of inducing local anesthesia include topical application, local tissue infiltration and nerve block.
- Topical application of anesthetic is helpful in nervous patients and children, and may be used before local tissue infiltration to lessen the discomfort of the injection.
- Addition of epinephrine (adrenaline) in injections retards the onset of anesthesia and increases its duration of action, so larger volumes of anesthetic can be used safely.
- The addition of epinephrine is unsuitable for use on digits or the penis, which are supplied by end arteries, because of the risk of inducing prolonged ischemia distal to the injection site.
- Injection techniques and regional sites for nerve blocks are best learned by supervised experience.
- Most minor procedures require 1–2 mL of anesthetic; a ring block should require a maximum of 3–5 mL.

The principal skin malignancies encountered in general practice are:
- basal cell carcinoma (BCC)
- squamous cell carcinoma (SCC)
- Bowen's disease (an in-situ variant of SCC)
- malignant melanoma (MM).

The benign lesions most often considered for surgery are:
- seborrheic keratoses
- viral warts
- melanocytic nevi
- dermatofibroma
- skin tags
- pyogenic granuloma.

Diagnosis of lesions

The ability to diagnose a lesion correctly is the most important skill a skin surgeon can acquire. Accurate diagnosis ensures that adequate surgical margins are included in the excision of malignant lesions, and conversely allows minimization of the margin of normal skin in the removal of benign lesions. Biopsy is very useful if the diagnosis is uncertain, and even experienced dermatological surgeons take biopsies before definitive excision if the diagnosis or the margins required are unclear. This text is not intended to provide the reader with an exhaustive knowledge of lesion recognition. More comprehensive works on the subject are listed in Further reading, page 114.

Patient history. In primary care, patients often present with a lesion that is causing them concern. Often, the lesion is a secondary reason for presentation or even an afterthought in a consultation for a separate problem. Taking a systematic patient history will aid diagnosis (Table 3.1).

Examination. After a history has been taken, the lesion and skin in general should be examined. Examination of the background skin may

TABLE 3.1

Questions to ask when taking a patient history

History	Significance
How long has the lesion been present?	Newly acquired lesions that persist for longer than 1 or 2 months may indicate neoplasm, particularly if the patient is in an older age group
Has a pigmented lesion changed in color or shape?	Alteration in shape or color may point towards malignancy
Has there been any bleeding?	Some benign lesions bleed, e.g. pyogenic granuloma and seborrheic keratoses. However, basal cell carcinomas may also bleed. In general, melanomas bleed only when well advanced, and in such cases the diagnosis is usually obvious
Does the lesion itch or hurt?	Squamous cell carcinomas are tender, particularly when squeezed. Benign nevi and seborrheic keratoses may also itch when irritated by clothing, etc.
Is there a history of occupational sun exposure, or has the patient lived or worked in the tropics?	Skin cancers in general are related to lifetime sun exposure. Malignant melanomas may be related to a single severe episode of sunburn
Is there a history of immunosuppressive drugs?	Immunosuppressive drugs increase the risk of skin cancer
Is there a family history of skin cancer?	This may indicate a genetic susceptibility, inherited skin type or conditions such as dysplastic nevus syndrome

show signs of chronic sun damage, such as dry, thickened, scaly skin with excess wrinkles. When examining the lesion, first assess your general impression – ask yourself 'Does this look benign?'. Check the lesion for pigment and, more importantly, any irregularity in the depth of color throughout (Figure 3.1). Note the presence of any tissue destruction, scabbing, evidence of bleeding or ulcer formation (Figures 3.2 and 3.3). Look at the edge of the lesion – is it regular and uniform (as in a benign nevus; Figure 3.4) or is there irregularity? Does the edge

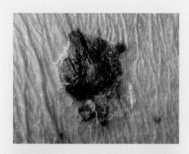

Figure 3.1 Malignant melanoma. Note the irregularity in color depth.

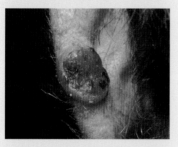

Figure 3.2 Squamous cell carcinoma showing gross ulceration and tissue destruction.

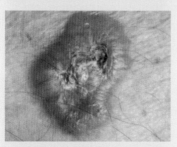

Figure 3.3 Basal cell carcinoma showing the typical pearly appearance, telangiectasia, raised rolled edge and central ulceration.

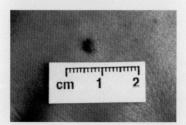

Figure 3.4 A benign nevus.

appear to invade the surrounding skin? Sometimes it is worth stretching the skin around a lesion, as other features, such as a rolled edge, may become apparent. It is also important to check for the presence of other lesions, particularly in sun-exposed areas.

Classification. Even if a definite diagnosis is not possible, lesions can often be classified as benign, pre-malignant or malignant. 'Pointers' towards the etiology of a lesion are shown in Table 3.2. If in doubt, err on the side of caution: assume the lesion is potentially malignant and take a biopsy.

Malignant skin lesions
An overview of malignant skin lesions is given below. For more details on the identification of skin malignancies, please refer to *Fast Facts: Skin Cancer*.

Basal cell carcinoma. BCCs are slow-growing, invasive, epithelial tumors arising from the basal layer of the epidermis. They are the most common

TABLE 3.2

Characteristics of benign versus potentially malignant lesions

Characteristic	Benign lesion	Potentially malignant lesion
Growth	Not growing	Growing
Bleeding	Absent	Present
Scabbing	No scab	Scab or keratin 'crust'
Number/location	Many other similar lesions	On a sun-exposed area of the body
Shape	Regular shape with smooth outline or line of symmetry	Irregular outline with no symmetry
Color	Uniform pigmentation	Variation in color throughout the lesion
Occurrence	Present for many years	New lesion

skin cancer, with 50% occurring on the head and neck, 30% on the upper trunk and the remainder on the limbs. BCCs vary in appearance, including a pearly papule (see Figure 3.3, page 29), a rodent ulcer (where the skin seems to have been 'nibbled' away [as if by a rodent], forming an ulcer), an erythematous scaling plaque on the trunk (Figure 3.5) and an infiltrating scar-like plaque (morpheic BCC; Figure 3.6). Occasionally, a BCC may be pigmented, resembling a melanoma.

Management. BCCs can cause extensive local destruction if left untreated but metastasis is an exceedingly rare event. As these tumors are generally slow growing, arranging treatment is not usually urgent. Several types of therapy are available. With proper patient and tumor selection, similar 10-year cure rates (of approximately 90%) are achievable with surgical excision, curettage and cautery, cryosurgery and radiotherapy.

Surgical excision. The margin of excision is normally 2–3 mm, or wider if the BCC has an aggressive histological pattern (e.g. micronodular, infiltrative or morpheic), is recurrent or large.

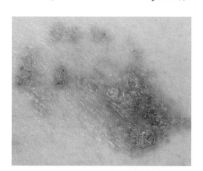

Figure 3.5 A thin, scaling plaque-like basal cell carcinoma with erythema, found on the trunk.

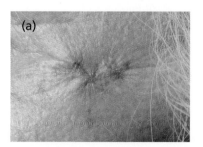
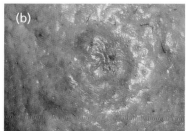

Figure 3.6 A morpheic basal cell carcinoma (a) with scar-like features; (b) presenting as an indurated plaque.

Curettage and cautery is a simple technique that can achieve good results in trained hands. It is appropriate for well-demarcated and relatively superficial tumors. Skill is required, not only in undertaking the technique, but also in selecting appropriate patients and tumors. It is not suited to recurrent tumors or those with aggressive histological patterns.

Cryosurgery is a skilled and specialized technique used mainly for well-defined superficial BCCs on the trunk. Histological confirmation is required before using this treatment. The timed spot-freeze technique is used to deliver a predetermined dose of liquid nitrogen to the lesion. Superficial BCCs generally require two 30-second freeze–thaw cycles to achieve a cure rate of 80–90%. The morbidity associated with this duration of freeze (e.g. pain, swelling and blistering) needs to be taken into account when planning treatment; surgical excision may cause less pain and/or scarring, although scarring is rare even with long freezes.

Radiotherapy has a role in the treatment of BCCs where surgery is likely to be very destructive (e.g. around the eyelid), when surgery is contraindicated or as a postoperative adjunctive therapy for aggressive tumors, especially if there is perineural spread. Multiple fractionated doses are required. It is generally restricted to patients over 60 years of age.

Topical imiquimod, a potent immunostimulant, has achieved histological clearance of superficial BCCs in controlled trials, with excellent cosmetic outcome. Results showed no histological evidence of residual tumor in 88% of lesions treated with a daily application for 6 weeks. Results were less impressive for nodular tumors. Practitioners need to be judicious in both tumor and patient selection. A pre-treatment biopsy is recommended. As this treatment is administered by the patient, the importance of complying with the full course of treatment should be explained. The 10-year cure rates are, as yet, unknown.

Photodynamic therapy (PDT) is a treatment option for carefully selected tumors, and is suitable for superficial BCC. Following topical application of a porphyrin-containing cream (Metvix®), intense light is shone on the area of application, which causes a reaction that destroys the cancerous cells. This process may need to be repeated 1–4 weeks after the first treatment session. PDT is generally only available in specialist centers.

Mohs' microscopically controlled surgery is used for tumors at high risk of recurrence and/or those arising at sites such as the eyelid or centrofacially where tissue conservation is important. Immediate examination of frozen sections of excised tissue allows histological confirmation of tumor clearance before wound closure and minimizes the removal of uninvolved tissue. Cure rates of up to 98% can be achieved. However, it is a time-consuming procedure requiring advanced training and specialist center infrastructure.

Squamous cell carcinoma. SCCs are the second most common type of skin cancer. They manifest as erythematous, scaling, proliferative lesions, which may grow over a period of several months. They may bleed easily and may be tender on palpation. SCCs occur predominantly in areas that have been heavily exposed to sunlight (head and neck, limbs and upper trunk). Up to 1% may metastasize, with a greater risk of secondary spread in lesions on the ear, lower lip and scalp (Figure 3.7). Patients with long-term immunosuppression are at increased risk of developing both primary SCCs and metastases.

Management. SCCs grow more rapidly than BCCs and should be treated as soon as is reasonable after the diagnosis is made or suspected. Treatment modalities include surgical excision and radiotherapy. Metastatic SCC from a primary cutaneous tumor should be treated initially with surgical excision, with or without radiotherapy. Cytotoxic chemotherapy may have a limited role in disseminated disease.

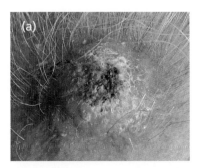 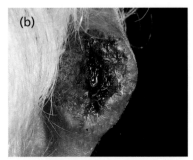

Figure 3.7 Invasive squamous cell carcinomas: (a) on the forehead and (b) on the ear.

Surgical excision is the treatment of choice for SCC. The margin of excision should be 3–5 mm around the clinical signs of the tumor.

Curettage and diathermy may be considered in patients with low-risk lesions.

Radiotherapy may be used for a primary tumor when surgery is likely to produce severe scarring or is unsuitable (e.g. for an elderly or infirm patient). Adjuvant radiotherapy may be used following excision of a high-risk primary tumor (e.g. a tumor with perineural spread on histopathology).

Investigation and follow-up of patients with primary SCC should be carried out every 6 months for at least 2 years after removal of a primary tumor. Clinical examination for signs of possible secondary tumor (e.g. in the regional lymph nodes) should be undertaken at each follow-up visit. Radiological, biochemical and hematological screening are not routine and are indicated only when there is evidence of metastatic disease on clinical examination.

Keratoacanthoma is probably a low-risk variant of SCC. It is a distinctive tumor, with a characteristic central keratin plug surrounded by erythematous skin (Figure 3.8).

Management. Surgical excision is the treatment of choice. Curettage and diathermy may be used if the diagnosis has been histologically confirmed.

Bowen's disease is the most common form of in-situ (intraepidermal) SCC. The prognosis for Bowen's disease is good, with approximately 5% progressing to invasive SCC over a number of years. It presents as a scaly, well-demarcated, erythematous plaque (Figure 3.9).

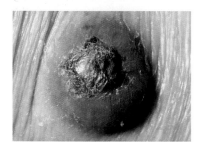

Figure 3.8 Keratoacanthoma, with a central keratin plug surrounded by erythematous skin.

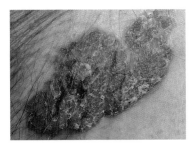

Figure 3.9 Bowen's disease presents as a well-demarcated, scaly, erythematous plaque.

Management. Diagnosis is confirmed by punch biopsy or, if the lesion is small enough, excision biopsy. If the lesion is excised, no further treatment is required besides sun-exposure counseling and a single follow-up appointment at 3 months to check the wound. If a biopsy was taken, the residual lesion will require treatment. Excision is not usually the treatment of choice as the individual lesions of Bowen's disease often present when they are already quite large. Topical therapy with 5-fluorouracil cream or imiquimod, or PDT is effective. Cryosurgery may be utilized by the experienced practitioner.

Melanoma is a malignant tumor derived from melanocytes. The most common site of involvement is the skin, although occasionally primary melanoma develops in other organs (eye, oral/nasal mucosa, vulval and anorectal mucosa). Melanomas are a major cause of premature death from cancer. Recognized risk factors are shown in Table 3.3.

TABLE 3.3
Risk factors for melanoma

- Personal or family history of melanoma
- Large numbers of nevi and/or dysplastic nevi
- Giant congenital melanocytic nevi
- Fair complexion
- Tendency to burn in the sun
- Sun-damaged skin
- History of non-melanoma skin cancer
- Immunodeficiency

The commonest sites for melanoma are the legs for women and the back for men (which are not the sites of greatest sun exposure). Early detection is associated with improved survival.

Any malignancy will grow irregularly and function abnormally. A melanoma produces pigment in abnormal amounts and elicits an immune response that will be reflected in the clinical appearance. A small but significant number of melanomas cannot be diagnosed on clinical appearance alone. A history of change may therefore be the only clue to the correct diagnosis.

Superficial spreading melanoma is the commonest type of melanoma, usually presenting as an irregularly pigmented macule (Figure 3.10).

Nodular melanoma is an aggressive tumor with an invasive growth pattern and can grow rapidly over weeks (see Figure 3.1, page 29). These tumors vary in color from black through red to amelanotic, and may defy the 'ABCD' rule (Table 3.4). The mnemonic EFG, which stands for 'elevated', 'firm' and 'growing for more than 1 month' is more appropriate. Nodular melanomas can be pedunculated, and may be mistaken for a hemangioma or a pyogenic granuloma.

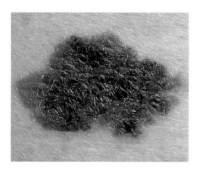

Figure 3.10 Superficial spreading melanoma, with characteristic asymmetry and irregular borders.

TABLE 3.4

Clinical features of melanoma – the ABCD rule

Asymmetry	One half of the lesion does not match the other
Border	Irregular, ragged, notched or blurred
Color	Multiple colors – not the same all over
Diameter	> 7 mm, or growing

Acral lentiginous melanoma is the most common form of melanoma in dark-skinned people; however, it is still a rare form of melanoma. It is seen on the palms, soles or nail bed. (Not all melanomas at these sites are of acral lentiginous type.)

Lentigo maligna (Hutchinson's melanotic freckle) is seen mostly on the face in elderly patients with sun-damaged skin (Figure 3.11). There is often a long delay before this type of in-situ melanoma becomes invasive. Patients will often be aware of these irregular, brown-to-black facial macules for many years. As such, they can be quite extensive at presentation even though still restricted to the epidermis. Distinction from benign lentigos may be impossible without histology. Invasive melanoma may arise within a lentigo maligna; this is described as a 'lentigo maligna melanoma'. Invasion can develop rapidly so excision is usually advised.

Desmoplastic melanoma is a rare and aggressive subtype of melanoma.

Management. If a diagnosis of melanoma cannot be confidently excluded on clinical grounds, the lesion should be excised or the patient referred for specialist opinion.

Surgical excision. Complete excision of the 'suspicious' lesion with a 2-mm lateral margin down to fat is recommended. Only sample a lesion by punch or shave biopsy if complete excision is difficult (e.g. a large, facial pigmented lesion), because a biopsy may not be representative of the lesion as a whole and it also alters the clinical appearance.

The initial excision of a suspicious pigmented lesion is a diagnostic procedure. It is done to exclude or confirm melanoma. Thus, a benign histology does not mean that the procedure was unnecessary.

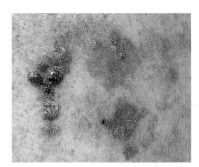

Figure 3.11 Lentigo maligna melanoma on a sun-damaged area of skin.

TABLE 3.5

Guidelines for melanoma excision margins

Melanoma	Margin
In situ (restricted to epidermis)	5 mm
< 1.5 mm thick	1 cm
1.5–4 mm thick	1 cm (min) to 2 cm (max)
> 4 mm thick	2 cm (min) to 3 cm (max)

If histology proves the lesion to be a melanoma then definitive surgical excision is needed. This should be explained to the patient before the initial excision.

Recommended excision margins are under constant review (Table 3.5). The main determinant is the tumor thickness, but margins may also vary according to anatomic site, patient, specific melanoma subtype and histological features. The depth of excision should equal the lateral margin where possible, but there is no need to excise beyond the deep fascia. Controversy surrounds the use of margins greater than 1 cm.

Radiotherapy has a role in the management of selected cases of primary melanoma (e.g. unresectable tumors and lentigo maligna if surgery is contraindicated). It may also be used as adjuvant therapy after surgery.

Management of metastasis requires referral to a melanoma unit or oncologist.

Benign skin lesions

Strategies for removing benign skin lesions include chemical and thermal cautery, curettage with or without cautery, shave excision, snip excision, liquid nitrogen cryosurgery, fine-wire diathermy, and simple incision and expression of cysts and abscesses. The preferred treatment options are shown in Table 3.6 (pages 40–1).

The surgical techniques required are discussed in Chapter 7. Choice of surgical technique is influenced by the nature of the lesion, its anatomic site and patient factors, which include skin color (cryosurgery is unsuitable for dark skin because of the risk of persistent depigmentation), propensity to unsightly scarring or keloid formation (see pages 49–50), and patient preference.

Seborrheic keratosis is a benign epidermal lesion that occurs with increasing frequency with age. The lesions are almost always multiple and have a characteristic 'stuck on' appearance (Figure 3.12). They vary from flesh-colored, through a range of browns, to a dark, almost black appearance. If scratched, they appear waxy.

Management. Operative intervention is made for diagnosis or because the patient is unhappy with the appearance or feel of the lesions. Cryosurgery, shave excision, electrodesiccation or curettage and cautery are all acceptable treatments. The authors prefer gentle curettage and chemical cautery.

Sebaceous hyperplasia. Each lesion is a small collection of sebaceous glands around a central follicle. They are papular umbilicated lesions, usually less than 6 mm in size, and have an off-white to yellow appearance (Figure 3.13). They are more common with advancing age and occur in areas with a high concentration of sebaceous glands, such as the nose, forehead and cheeks.

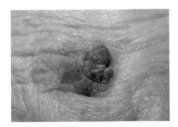

Figure 3.12 Seborrheic keratosis. Note the 'stuck on' appearance.

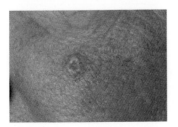

Figure 3.13 Sebaceous hyperplasia shows as a white/yellow waxy lesion.

TABLE 3.6

Preferred treatment options for benign skin lesions

Condition	Treatment			
	Curettage	Shave	Excision	Cryosurgery
Seborrheic keratosis	++	+	X	++
Viral wart	+	–	X	++
Skin tags				
Narrow-necked	X	++	X	+
Wide-necked, fibro-epithelial polyp	–	++	X	–
Dermatofibroma (histiocytoma)	X	X	–	X
Pyogenic granuloma	++	++	+	++
Cherry angioma (Campel de Morgan spot)	X	X	X	+
Venous lakes	X	X	–	++
Lipoma	X	X	++	X
Epidermoid cyst	X	X	++	X
Milia	X	X	X	X
Sebaceous hyperplasia	–	X	–	X
Actinic (solar) keratosis	+	+	–	++
Nevus				
Non-pigmented	X	++	+	X
Pigmented, benign (raised)	X	++	–	X
Pigmented, benign (flat)	X	+	+	X
Hairy, benign	X	+	++	X
'Suspicious' or changing	X	–	++	X
Keloid	X	X	X	X
Chondrodermatitis nodularis chronica helicis	–	–	++	–

++, acceptable treatment (preferred); +, acceptable treatment, second choice; –, treatment not usually used for this lesion; X, not acceptable. BCC, basal cell carcinoma; R, reassurance of patient is a viable alternative to treatment.

Special considerations

R

R, or topical treatment with salicylic/lactic acid

R, snip excision, treatment with cautery as 'hot scalpel'
R, treatment with cautery as 'hot scalpel'

R, once the diagnosis is explained to patients they are
usually satisfied with no treatment

Cryosurgery should be performed only when there has been prior
histological confirmation of the diagnosis

R, fine-wire diathermy is the treatment of choice if
intervention is required

R

R

R

R, if treatment is required, puncture and express the contents and cyst wall

R, excision biopsy if clinical suspicion of BCC. Fine-wire diathermy is effective

R, 5-fluorouracil cream, excision of thick lesions with active base
indicated to exclude malignant transformation

R
R
R, shave or excision not usually necessary if benign diagnosis confident –
resultant scar may have worse appearance than the lesion

R, shave excision may leave some of the mole and hair follicles behind

Specialist referral is ideal when the cosmetic outcome is important.
Accurate clinical diagnosis may negate the need for biopsy in over
50% of cases

Principal treatment is intralesional injection of steroid. Specialist referral if
indicated

R, sculpture of the underlying damaged cartilage to remove rough edges

Management. Sebaceous hyperplasia may be difficult to distinguish from a small BCC, and in such cases biopsy is indicated. These lesions are benign and do not require treatment; they may respond to cryosurgery or fine-wire diathermy but are usually too deep.

Milia are small lesions (1–3 mm) with a white, papular appearance (Figure 3.14). They are small cystic structures that either connect directly to the skin surface or arise within a sweat duct or hair follicle. They commonly occur on the face in patients of any age and are benign.

Management. Surgical treatment is indicated only for cosmetic reasons. The least invasive technique is to puncture the overlying skin with a sterile needle and to express the contents and cyst wall using a comedone extractor or digital pressure.

Molluscum contagiosum is a viral infection of the skin that appears as small, wart-like swellings. More common in children, it spreads by skin to skin contact or by sharing towels or clothes.

Management. Although swellings are best left to heal naturally, the healing can be quickened by squeezing the swellings to empty out the infected contents. Curettage, cryotherapy and diathermy are all possible treatment options, but are not recommended in children.

Actinic (solar) keratosis develops in sun-damaged skin and occurs with increasing frequency with age. The individual lesion may be flat and irregularly shaped with an adherent scale (Figure 3.15); some may develop a thick keratinous plaque or even a cutaneous horn.

Solar keratoses are closely related to skin type and have a higher incidence in outdoor workers, pale-skinned individuals living in tropical

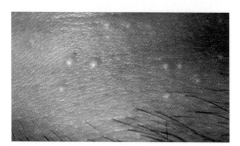

Figure 3.14 Milia are small, white papular lesions.

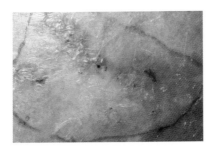

Figure 3.15 Actinic (solar) keratosis is a scaly patch on sun-damaged skin.

climates and sun-worshippers. Their appearance is a sign of overexposure to the damaging effects of solar radiation in susceptible individuals.

These lesions are pre-malignant. Transformation into invasive SCC occurs at a very low rate, though the rate is much greater in immunocompromised patients. More important than the risk of an individual lesion turning into an invasive SCC is the fact that solar keratoses are markers of solar damage and persons are at risk of developing BCC, SCC or melanoma elsewhere on their skin. A complete skin examination is therefore essential.

To distinguish solar keratosis from SCC or BCC, it is useful to remove any surface scale to inspect the base of the lesion. The remainder of the sun-exposed skin may show solar elastosis or lentigines, with increased wrinkles and a general dryness and thickening. This is described as 'field change'.

Management. The patient should be warned of the risks of further sun exposure and advised on early detection of skin cancer.

Treatment depends on the thickness of the lesion, the number of lesions present and their cosmetic appearance. Thin, non-'suspicious' lesions may be observed, but if treatment is required cryosurgery, curettage, 5-fluorouracil cream, imiquimod or PDT are all acceptable. Thicker lesions may require cryosurgery. Those with clinical features of transformation should be biopsied. Multiple thinner lesions are best treated with 5-fluorouracil cream, imiquimod or cryosurgery.

Dermatofibroma is a benign dermal tumor. Most cases are solitary, though multiple lesions may occur. They are more common on the lower limbs, and women are affected more than men. There is sometimes a history of minor trauma or an insect bite followed by the rapid growth of the tumor to its usual size of 5–10 mm.

Examination of the lesion reveals a hard nodule attached to the overlying skin, which may exhibit a brown discoloration (Figure 3.16). The tumor consists mainly of collagen, which is tightly packed and gives the tumor its characteristic 'hard' feel. The tumor may extend through the dermis and into the subcuticular fat but is unattached to underlying fascia. If the lesion is compressed, there is a dimpling of the skin over the lesion.

Management. Reassurance of the patient is usually all that is required. If the lesion itches or is tender, the patient may request removal. As the lesion extends through the thickness of the dermis, surgical treatment involves excision of the lesion down to the subcutaneous fat layer. However, only a small lateral margin is required.

Pyogenic granuloma is a common vascular tumor that usually presents as a soft, friable, bleeding papule, 5–10 mm in size (Figure 3.17). There is often a history of preceding minor trauma followed by a rapidly growing lesion that bleeds easily. The tumor is mainly comprised of granulation tissue covered by a flattened epidermis. The capillary

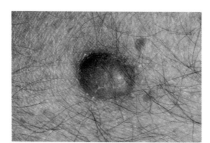

Figure 3.16 Dermatofibroma is a hard, benign, dermal nodule attached to the overlying skin.

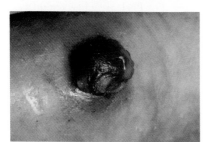

Figure 3.17 Pyogenic granuloma is a rapidly growing vascular tumor.

network of the granulation tissue is prominent, which explains its coloration and ease of bleeding.

Management. Treatment should be curettage and cautery. It is important to obtain pathological confirmation of the diagnosis, because a rapid-growing, nodular, malignant melanoma may resemble a pyogenic granuloma. The recurrence rate following curettage is low. Recurrent lesions, where the diagnosis has prior histological confirmation, may be treated with cryosurgery.

Viral warts occur on any area of the skin, as well as on mucous membranes. The causal agent is the human papilloma virus, many subtypes of which have now been identified. Many warts involute spontaneously within 2 years or so, but some may persist even after vigorous treatment. Recent evidence shows that occlusion of warts with duct tape may be an effective and relatively painless treatment.

Verruca vulgaris (common wart) presents as a firm hyperkeratotic nodule more commonly on the hands, though they may occur anywhere on the skin (Figure 3.18).

Management. Some patients may accept reassurance alone. If treatment is requested, topical paints such as salicylic acid are first-line treatment. If these do not work, cryosurgery is effective, though multiple treatments, usually 3 weeks apart, may be required.

Verruca plana (flat or plane wart) presents as a slightly elevated smooth papule, 1–3 mm in size. They are usually multiple and occur preferentially on the dorsum of the hands and on the face.

Management. Treatment can be difficult. Topical skin irritants such as retinoid creams may be tried. Paints are difficult to apply precisely because the warts are very small. Cryosurgery may lead to

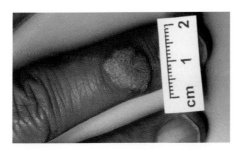

Figure 3.18 Verruca vulgaris (common viral wart).

postinflammatory hypo- or hyperpigmentation of surrounding skin for similar reasons. Ultimately, these lesions resolve spontaneously without scarring, and thus reassurance is often the best treatment.

Verruca plantaris (verruca) occurs on the soles of the feet and is common at points of pressure, such as the ball and heel of the foot. The area of skin affected appears thickened and black dots (thrombosed capillaries) are apparent beneath. They are often painful because of the effect of the thickened epidermis on the pressure points of the foot.

Management. Treatment is as for common warts, but it is helpful to pare away the thickened epidermis before cryosurgery or application of paints. Many lesions are difficult to treat, and without treatment most lesions persist for years.

Condylomata acuminata (genital warts) occur on the genital area, anus and perineum.

Management. Genital warts may be treated by cryosurgery, snip excision, podophyllin paint or imiquimod cream. These lesions may be pre-malignant and it is therefore important to emphasize the need for regular cervical Pap smears to affected women and partners of affected men, even if they are asymptomatic.

Skin tags (acrochordons) are common lesions that occur more frequently with advancing age and are more prevalent in overweight people. They may occur on any skin surface but are more common in the axilla, around the neck and in the groin. Larger similar lesions are termed fibro-epitheliomatous polyps. Both lesions are fibromas with a connective tissue stalk and a hyperkeratotic dermis.

Management is by snip excision, cryosurgery or cautery excision.

Melanocytic nevi (moles) are localized collections of melanocytes in the dermis and epidermis.

- Junctional nevi are lesions in which melanocytes are confined to the epidermis and dermal–epidermal junction, and are usually flat pigmented macules.
- Compound nevi – raised, pigmented papules – have melanocytes at both the dermal–epidermal junction and deeper in the dermis.

- Intradermal nevi – non-pigmented papules – have melanocytes only within the dermis and have no associated epidermal or junctional component.

The majority of moles are induced by sunlight in people predisposed to their development. The risk of a benign mole turning into a melanoma is very low, and prophylactic excision to prevent malignant transformation is not recommended. However, large numbers of moles, both common acquired and dysplastic nevi, are markers of increased risk for the development of melanoma elsewhere on the skin.

Congenital nevi are not always visible at birth. Many only become apparent in the first year of life (Figure 3.19). They can be classified by diameter, as:

- small < 15 mm
- medium 15–200 mm
- large > 200 mm.

Incidence in Caucasians is approximately 1% and the nevi are mostly small. Giant congenital nevi affect only 1 in 500 000 babies. Melanoma may develop in congenital nevi. The lifetime risk of melanoma arising in a large congenital nevus is controversial, but is probably 4–6%. The risk associated with small and medium nevi is negligible.

Management. Routine excision of all congenital nevi to prevent melanoma development is not recommended.

Dysplastic nevi (atypical moles) are strikingly variable. They are 10 mm or more in diameter, irregular in outline, a haphazard mixture of tan, black and pink, and flat with a small palpable dermal component (Figure 3.20). An erythematous margin is common. In short, they look like melanomas. The term 'dysplastic' is a misnomer as histological dysplasia is not always present and is not required for a diagnosis.

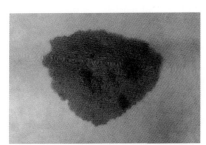

Figure 3.19 A congenital nevus.

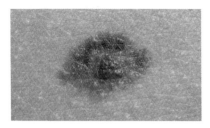

Figure 3.20 A dysplastic nevus with an irregular outline and pigment variation.

Dysplastic nevi are commonly familial and in some families are markers of increased melanoma risk. Even in families without melanoma, dysplastic nevi are an independent risk factor for development of melanoma elsewhere on the skin.

Management. If any doubt exists clinically about the nature of a lesion, an excision biopsy should be performed or the patient should be referred to a dermatologist. If a patient presents with one or more dysplastic nevi, the entire skin surface should be examined carefully. The patient should be given advice about early detection of skin cancer and how to minimize the harmful effects of sun exposure. In patients with multiple lesions or a family history of melanoma, baseline clinical photographs will help to identify changes in existing moles or to detect new ones. Review arrangements are a matter for the individual clinician; however, high-risk patients should be followed up for their lifetime.

Acquired nevi are very common. A patient may request the removal of a nevus for cosmetic reasons, because it is catching in clothes or jewelry, or because of a change within it.

Management. The most appropriate surgical management is shave excision or excision and primary closure. The former may, however, leave behind some pigment and hair follicles, but conversely may result in a superior scar. All moles should be sent for histology. As well as detecting an early melanoma with banal clinical features, it may also avoid the risk of litigation at a later stage if a patient develops metastatic melanoma with an undetected primary lesion. Even if the metastases were unrelated to the lesion excised, this would be impossible to prove without histology.

Chondrodermatitis nodularis chronica helicis (CNCH) is characterized by a painful nodule, most commonly on the helix of the ear

(Figure 3.21). The patient complains of pain when pressure is exerted on the area (e.g. when trying to sleep). The condition most frequently affects men over 40 and there may be a history of outdoor work or exposure to cold. Lesions occur less commonly on the tragus or antihelix. The lesion tends to be oval, inflamed and appears fixed to the underlying cartilage. The cause of this lesion is unclear but it has been postulated that relatively poor circulation to the cartilage predisposes it to pressure necrosis during sleep.

Management. Attempted extrusion of the necrotic cartilage through the skin leads to an overlying inflamed nodule. Most lesions will resolve if the patient can be persuaded to sleep on the other side. Special pillows that alleviate local pressure may also help. Intralesional injection of triamcinolone has a 20–30% success rate and is worth a try. Surgical excision of the nodule will lead to recurrence unless any irregularity of the cartilage is smoothed out. Some skin surgeons recommend the use of cryosurgery, particularly in early small lesions.

Hypertrophic scarring and keloids are caused by a proliferation of fibrous tissue in damaged skin as a result of surgery, immunization, acne, etc. (Figure 3.22). Wound infection and dehiscence of surgical

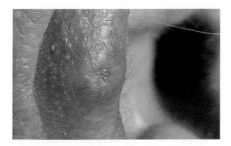

Figure 3.21
Chondrodermatitis nodularis chronica helicis, a painful benign nodule on the helix of the ear.

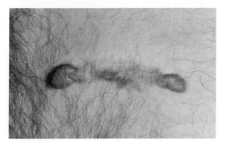

Figure 3.22 Keloid formation in a previous surgical scar.

scars predispose to healing with hypertrophy. Keloids may form at any site, but are more common in the upper body and tend to be more vigorous in the young and those with pigmented skin. The lesions are firm and may be slightly tender or itchy; they are raised from the skin and may grow beyond the boundaries of the initial skin insult. A previous keloid scar indicates a susceptibility to the formation of further keloids in wounded skin, and cosmetic surgery should be avoided in patients with a history of keloid formation.

Management. Standard treatment for both hypertrophic scarring and keloids is intralesional steroid injection, which usually needs to be repeated several times. Laser therapy, cryosurgery and surgical excision of scars are also widely practiced, but outcomes are unpredictable. The best results are achieved by clinicians who specialize in this area.

Key points – lesion identification and management

- Accurate diagnosis is essential to ensure adequate surgical margins in the excision of malignant lesions and minimization of margins in the removal of benign lesions.
- Biopsy is very useful if the diagnosis is uncertain.
- Basal cell carcinoma (BCC) is the most common skin cancer and is usually slow-growing; metastasis is extremely rare.
- Squamous cell carcinoma grows more rapidly than BCC and should be treated as soon as is reasonable after diagnosis; surgical excision is the treatment of choice.
- Early detection of melanomas is associated with improved survival; a history of change may be the only clue to the correct diagnosis.
- Actinic (solar) keratoses, dysplastic nevi and large numbers of nevi are all risk factors for malignant lesions elsewhere; a complete skin examination is essential in patients with these lesions.
- Condylomata acuminata (genital warts) may be pre-malignant, so the importance of regular cervical Pap smears should be emphasized to affected women and partners of affected men, even if they are asymptomatic.

Remember, all surgery causes scarring. The stages in planning successful treatment are discussed in this chapter and are shown in Figure 4.1. Factors that must be considered before embarking on surgery include:

- diagnosis
- necessity
- cosmetics and regional anatomy
- potential complications
- comorbidity/drugs
- surgical technique and aftercare.

Diagnosis

If a working or differential diagnosis is not made, then a surgical plan cannot be formulated. The ability to recognize lesions with confidence and knowing what to do having made the diagnosis, are the most important and difficult aspects of skin surgery.

Necessity

When a diagnosis has been made, the need for an operative procedure can be assessed. The removal of a benign lesion can be justified only if it is in a cosmetically unimportant position or if removal is necessary because of irritation or repeated trauma. In cosmetically sensitive areas, removal of benign lesions should be undertaken with the utmost care; referral to experts may be deemed necessary by either you or the patient. There is no point in removing benign lesions yourself if the patient requests excision by a plastic surgeon, because such patients are likely to be intolerant of even a minor complication.

Cosmetics

A number of factors, including the skill of the surgeon, influence the final cosmetic result. It is important to use the correct surgical technique for the condition to be treated and to use the least invasive method available.

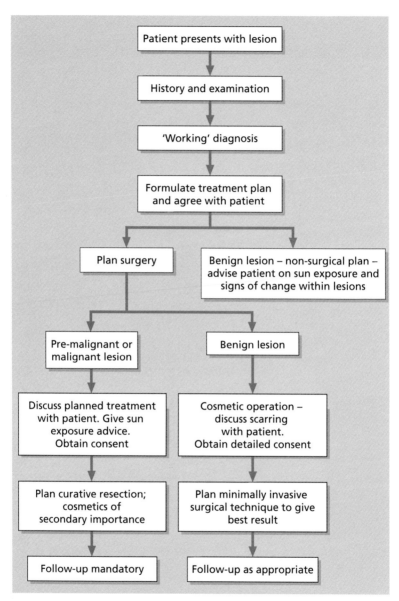

Figure 4.1 Planning a successful treatment.

Site. Some sites produce notoriously poor cosmetic results; for example, surgery on the upper trunk may leave a hyperemic or keloid scar (see pages 49–50).

Skin tension and the orientation of the incision may affect the final
result. Skin tension lines are the lines of preferred orientation of
wounds and take into account lines of least skin tension and skin folds
(which usually follow skin tension lines). In a given area of skin, there
may be more than one tension line. Skin tension lines are generated by
a number of factors, including:

- the orientation of underlying muscle groups
- fibrous bands between the dermis and underlying muscle groups
- joint mobility
- gravity.

A wound made at 90° to the lines of maximum tension will tend to
spring open (Figure 4.2a). Wound edges of an incision oblique to the
tension lines will tend to 'slip'; in Figure 4.2b the wound edges have
slipped because of uneven tension. If a wound is planned in this oblique
manner, it is useful to place perpendicular skin markings across the

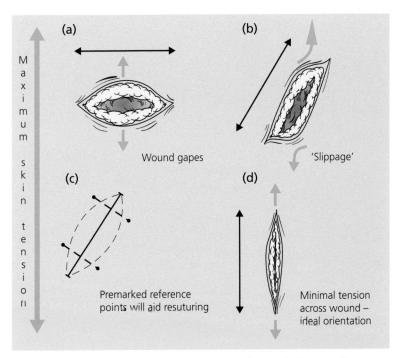

Figure 4.2 Skin tension lines and orientation of wounds (see text for
explanation).

planned incision, making it easier to suture and avoid a dog-ear
(Figure 4.2c). An incision along the line of maximum skin tension will
tend to have the least tension across the wound, making approximation
of the edges easier and the final scar less liable to splay with time
(Figure 4.2d).

Occasionally there may be good reason to use an alternative
orientation, for example if:

- a skin fold can be used to conceal a scar that does not run along a
  tension line
- the lesion lies across an area of high skin mobility, such as an
  underlying joint
- the long axis of a lesion lies across the tension lines.

Identifying skin tension lines. In general, skin tension is predictable;
the preferred incision lines are illustrated in Figure 4.3. It is worth
assessing skin tension by compression. If the area is compressed in the

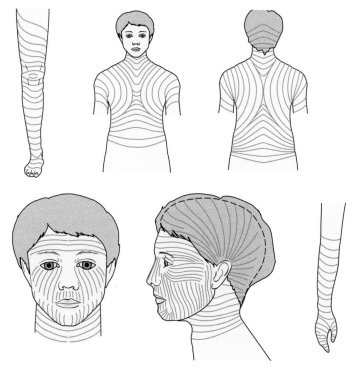

Figure 4.3 Preferred incision lines.

direction of planned surgery, the skin will wrinkle easily across the lines of maximum tension and the operator will feel the skin moving readily. Minimal wrinkling occurs and skin movement is less along the tension lines (Figure 4.4).

Size of the incision is also significant – larger incisions leave larger scars. The amount of tissue removed also influences the final result; for example, a potential space may be created by the removal of a cyst and this may leave a dimple if the space is not closed.

Sutures. The type of suture used is important. Absorbable sutures or silk used to close a wound superficially may initiate an inflammatory response; they also absorb fluids and potentially bacteria, increasing the risk of wound contamination. Using an inappropriately large-bore suture (e.g. a 3-0 on the face), will leave a laddered effect. Leaving sutures in place for too long before removal produces the same problem.

Suture technique is also important. In a wound under tension, if buried sutures are not used the wound edges may migrate or the wound may dehisce. The resultant scar will be wide and hyperemic. Everting the wound edges with mattress sutures will produce a superior result in some sites.

Postoperative factors. Postoperative infection will increase scarring and may cause dehiscence. Heavy manual work immediately after an

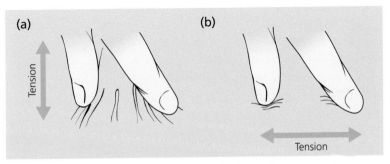

Figure 4.4 (a) If skin is compressed across the lines of maximum skin tension, wrinkling occurs. (b) If compressed along the tension lines, less wrinkling and movement occurs.

operation may open wounds on the trunk or limbs. Inadequate dressing of the wound postoperatively may predispose to infection. Appropriate aftercare is therefore essential.

Skin anatomy and scar formation

Skin surgery has the potential to cause unsightly scarring. Careful planning and use of the correct surgical techniques will reduce this. Minimally invasive techniques such as shave excision or curettage produce scars that are cosmetically more acceptable and minimize the risk of complications.

A basic knowledge of the anatomy of the skin (Figure 4.5) and scar formation will aid the surgeon in the planning stage. The thickness of the skin and its component parts vary according to the body site. The dermis is thickest on the back and the epidermis is thickest on the palms and soles. This variation has important consequences for healing rates and will affect the choice of surgical technique.

Healing by secondary intention. If a procedure removes only the epidermis and the dermal–epidermal junction is not breached, as with gentle curettage, the resulting erosion usually heals without any visible scar. A scar forms only if the dermal–epidermal junction is penetrated. Wounds left to heal by secondary intention undergo contraction, inflammation, formation of granulation tissue and finally re-epithelialization; all of these factors influence the appearance and function of the resultant scar. For example, contraction on the lower eyelid may produce an ectropion (where the lower eyelid is turned out, exposing the cornea to potential damage), while contraction on the lower third of the nose can lead to tenting of the nostril. In contrast, healing by secondary intention often works well on the bridge of the nose. Other sites that are suitable for healing by secondary intention are shown in Figure 4.6.

The wound depth will also influence the scar. Superficial wounds may re-epithelialize from the appendageal structures rather than the wound edges. This hastens the healing process and the resultant scar is usually flat or minimally depressed, with slight hypopigmentation. Deep wounds that destroy or remove the skin appendages are slower to heal

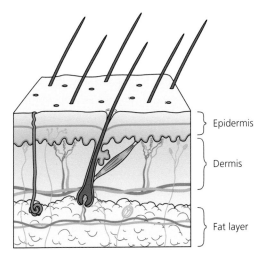

Figure 4.5 Basic anatomy of the skin. The epidermis is a thin (0.1–1.4 mm thick) cover of stratified squamous epithelium. The subcutaneous fat layer is comprised of loose connective tissue and fat. It is present in all areas of the skin and, like the dermis, varies in thickness. The important layer in terms of surgery is the dermis, a supportive matrix of connective tissue including, in the deep dermis, the collagen that gives the skin its tensile strength and the skin appendages. If the deep dermis is wounded (surgically), scarring is inevitable. If an area of dermis is lost, the resultant scar is devoid of appendages and will appear flat and featureless.

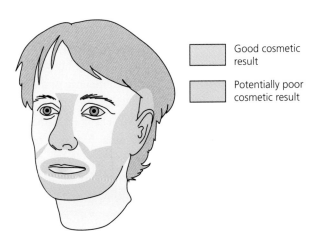

Figure 4.6 Suitability of sites for healing by secondary intention.

by secondary intention than superficial ones. Re-epithelialization occurs at the rate of 1 cm per month from the wound edges. The resultant scar is atrophic, pale and devoid of skin appendages. This wound-healing process involves a number of stages. Initially, the wound fills with clot. This results in a fibrin network through which granulation tissue permeates, producing a structure that fibroblasts migrate along. The collagen in the dermis contracts, making the wound smaller, and epithelialization occurs from the wound edges. This process takes longer than secondary intention healing of a superficial wound, but nonetheless may give a comparable cosmetic result to primary closure in carefully selected sites (see Figure 4.6).

Healing by primary closure. A clean wound with well-defined edges is required – most scalpel excisions are suitable. The edges of the wound are apposed to realign the skin structures and held in place with sterile skin-closure strips, sutures, staples, tissue adhesive or clips. Healing is complex and occurs in three stages.

The inflammatory phase is the first stage in which platelets, macrophages and leukocytes invade the wound, leading to the formation of a clot in the wound defect. The epithelial cells of the epidermis start to migrate along the cut edge of the dermis, and kinins are released, leading to a hyperemic reaction in the tissue immediately surrounding the wound. Fibroblasts initiate collagen synthesis within the first 48 hours. This phase lasts approximately 5 days.

The proliferative phase is the next stage of wound repair and begins at about 4–6 days. There is intense proliferation of fibroblasts, and capillaries continue to proliferate under the influence of the kinins. Fibroblasts migrate along fibrin strands, which are now vertically oriented within the wound. The epidermal cells unite in the upper dermis and the epidermis thickens in this area. A crust is formed on the wound surface, and late in the proliferative phase, at about 10–12 days, collagen is laid down by the fibroblasts, increasing the tensile strength of the wound. Because the fibroblasts are aligned vertically within the wound, the collagen is initially laid down in this direction. This vertical alignment and subsequent contracture has great significance in the eventual appearance of the wound (Figure 4.7).

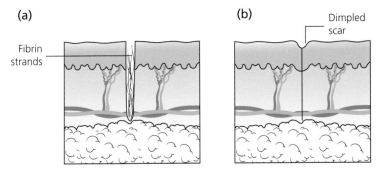

(a)

Fibrin
strands

(b)

Dimpled
scar

Figure 4.7 Vertical wound contraction. (a) Initial wound; (b) contraction.

The maturation phase is the final stage, beginning at about
2 weeks and lasting for many years after surgery. Remodeling of the
collagen within the dermis occurs along the lines of tension, leading
to a gradual increase in the tensile strength of the wound. Vascular
changes reduce during the first 12 months and the redness of the scar
fades. Nerve growth continues slowly, and remodeling of the collagen
adds strength and 'flattens' out the scar with time. Scar tissue never
reaches the tensile strength of unwounded skin and may be as little as
20% of the strength of normal skin at 2–3 weeks. Because of this poor
strength, it is advisable to insert buried dermal reabsorbable sutures to
allow the wound to heal in approximation and to minimize splaying.

Key points – treatment planning

- All surgery causes scarring.
- A benign lesion should only be removed if it is in a cosmetically
  unimportant position or if removal is necessary because of
  irritation or repeated trauma.
- In general, an incision along the line of maximum skin tension
  will tend to have the least tension across the wound, so that the
  final scar is less liable to splay with time.
- If the incision does not breach the dermal–epidermal junction
  (e.g. gentle curettage), the resulting erosion usually heals
  without any visible scar.

All surgeons experience complications. Good surgeons forewarn patients of potential problems, minimize the risks and deal promptly with any complications that arise. Accurate audit using surgical logbooks will allow easy identification of complications and surgical practices that require modification and improvement.

Regional anatomy

The surgeon should be aware of the regional anatomy of underlying structures. A number of important structures run superficially and may be damaged during skin surgery. In areas of the body such as the nose, ears, lower leg, palms, soles and digits, there is little laxity in the surrounding skin, making wound closure difficult or impossible.

Knowledge of problem areas is vital to minimize complications (Figure 5.1).

Head and neck. The skin of the head and neck tends to be thin, with little subcuticular fat. Muscles, nerves and blood vessels in some areas

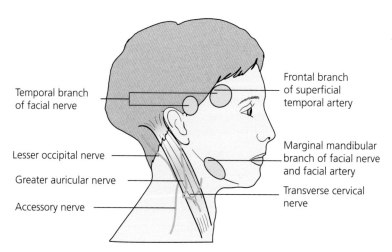

Temporal branch of facial nerve

Frontal branch of superficial temporal artery

Lesser occipital nerve

Marginal mandibular branch of facial nerve and facial artery

Greater auricular nerve

Accessory nerve

Transverse cervical nerve

Figure 5.1 Danger areas in the head and neck.

are only millimeters below the skin surface. Identification of these areas allows surgery to be planned more carefully. A useful technique is to use large volumes of diluted anesthetic to 'puff up' the skin just deep to the dermis, thereby creating an artificially thickened subcuticular fat layer that affords the deep structures more protection (Figure 5.2).

Superficial temporal artery and facial artery. The important superficial blood vessels of the head and neck are the superficial temporal artery (notably the frontal branch) and the facial artery. The superficial temporal artery is most vulnerable as it crosses the temple. The branches are usually palpable at this point. The artery emerges from behind the parotid immediately in front of the external auditory meatus and remains superficial as it ascends vertically towards the temple. Accidental transection of this artery is important only from a hemostatic point of view, as there is adequate crossover blood flow from the opposite side and other blood vessels. Transection of larger branches should be dealt with by tying off the offending vessel, as these arteries tend to be large and cautery alone may not provide adequate hemostasis.

Supraorbital and supratrochlear vessels and nerves are potentially endangered during surgery on medial forehead areas. The facial artery is palpable approximately halfway along the mandible, at which point it is a useful landmark for the marginal mandibular branch of the facial nerve. The facial artery is fairly deep at this point, but care should be taken when operating on thin patients or during excision of a deep tumor.

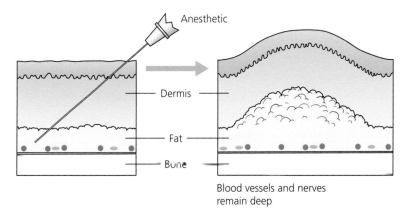

Figure 5.2 'Puffing up' the skin with anesthetic to protect deep structures.   61

The great vessels in the neck are protected by overlying muscles and should not present a problem in skin surgery. The external jugular vein and its tributaries may be prominent, particularly in thin patients, and care should be taken.

Facial nerve. This nerve innervates all the muscles of facial expression. It emerges from the stylomastoid foramen and enters the parotid almost immediately. When it emerges from the parotid, it has already split into its major branches. These then have a superficial course until they penetrate deeply to innervate their target muscles. Transection of a branch will result in paralysis of the target muscle and facial asymmetry.

The temporal branch of the facial nerve is responsible for raising the eyebrow. It is vulnerable where it emerges from the parotid and crosses over the zygomatic arch. It remains superficial up into the region of the temple. The combination of its superficial course, the thin subcuticular fat layer and the underlying bony prominences contribute to the danger of surgery in this area.

The marginal mandibular branch of the facial nerve may have a superficial course, particularly in elderly patients, as it crosses the mandible near the facial artery (see previously).

The cervical branch of the facial nerve and the spinal accessory nerve have a superficial course in the neck. The cervical branch of the facial nerve is protected by the platysma muscle, but in the elderly this may be paper-thin and as such the nerve may be exposed accidentally. The nerve is vulnerable about midway along the sternocleidomastoid muscle, approximately 6.5 cm below the external auditory meatus (a circle with a radius of 3.5 cm around this point covers the danger area). The spinal accessory nerve emerges into the posterior cervical triangle from deep to the sternocleidomastoid about two-thirds of the way down the muscle. Damage to the spinal accessory nerve may result in an inability to elevate the shoulder.

Facial features. Other important considerations in the head and neck are the facial features. In general, it is difficult to achieve a satisfactory cosmetic outcome when tension is applied in areas with a free edge, such as the nostrils, lower eyelid and vermilion border (the margin between the skin of the face and the skin of the lip) because of notching or ectropion (where the lower eyelid is turned out, exposing the cornea to potential damage). Even for relatively small excisions, cutaneous flaps and grafts are often required in these areas to remove tension from the free edge. For this reason, it is suggested that only experienced surgeons perform head and neck surgery.

Eyelids. Surgery to the eyelids is extremely difficult because of the thin skin and delicate muscle fibers. Surgery on, or adjacent to, the lower lid needs to be carefully planned to avoid tension from wound closure or subsequent contracture. In the elderly, this is particularly important as the tension of the lower lid is reduced and minimal contracture can cause an ectropion.

Nose. The nasolacrimal duct is situated superficially for only a few millimeters below its origin near to the medial canthus. The skin of the upper nose is quite mobile, whereas the skin of the lower nose is sebaceous and adherent to the underlying cartilage. Surgery to the lower area is difficult and large defects cannot be closed.

Lips. The vermilion border is extremely important cosmetically and if it is incised it is important to realign it accurately.

Hands and feet. The skin of the palm and the sole is thick, with little spare tissue. Surgery on these areas is difficult and the scope for wound closure should be assessed before any procedure. Healing by secondary intention is not desirable in these areas as it may be associated with wound contraction, leading to irregular and often tender scars (see pages 56–8). If primary closure is not easily achievable, then specialist referral for consideration of a flap or graft is advised.

Shins. The skin overlying the anterior shin has little laxity. In elderly patients and those with edema, the perfusion of this area is often poor and healing may be slow and complicated by ulceration. Again, in the elderly, particularly women, the dermis may be thin and fragile, preventing insertion of dermal-buried sutures – this may compromise closure.

An important anatomic 'hot spot' in this region is the path of the common peroneal nerve as it winds around the neck of the fibula. Accidental section of this nerve leads to foot drop.

Joints. Surgery around joints should be planned carefully as the mobility of the skin in these areas may put tension across a wound. This can be minimized by correct orientation of the incision (see pages 53–4).

Infection

This can be expected in 2–4% of minor surgical procedures conducted in an office setting. Obviously, it is more common in 'dirty' operations, such as surgery for ulcerated skin cancers or abscesses, and prophylactic antibiotic therapy may be indicated in such cases. It is important to recognize infection early and to take appropriate steps. Treatment with a broad-spectrum antibiotic with good coverage of penicillin-resistant staphylococci is required. Any pus should be evacuated, and in severe cases sutures should be removed and the wound left to heal by secondary intention.

Bleeding

Excess blood loss can occur during or after a procedure. During an operation, bleeding can be controlled by pressure, cautery or by tying off offending blood vessels. Rarely, a drainage tube is required. Bleeding after a procedure can usually be controlled by application of firm pressure to a wound. Occasionally, a hematoma will form and the wound may need to be opened, drained and re-sutured once hemostasis is achieved.

Nerve damage

Cutaneous sensory nerve damage will occur when the skin is cut, rendering a small area anesthetic. This is not usually a problem, as overlapping sensory innervation of the skin is the norm and sensory loss usually diminishes with time. If there is evidence of persistent motor-nerve damage, for example facial or digital nerve damage that is not simply a product of the anesthetic administered, then urgent referral to a specialist center is indicated.

Tendon damage

This should not occur in minor skin surgery. If it is evident following a procedure, however, prompt referral is indicated.

Wound dehiscence

A wound may split open if:
- the wound edges are under too much tension
- there is secondary wound infection
- sutures are removed too early.

Wounds do not achieve full strength for many weeks or months after surgery. They are vulnerable in the first few weeks after removal of the sutures, and patients should be instructed to curtail physical activities that stress wounds. Early dehiscences can be re-sutured, while late dehiscences are often best left to heal by secondary intention. Some patients have tissue-thin skin and the sutures cut through as soon as they are pulled together. In such cases, pulley or mattress sutures can be tried, taking deep bites. Sometimes the wound will have to be taped and left to heal by secondary intention.

Scarring

Splayed scarring is most common on the back and is almost unavoidable. Deep slow-absorbing sutures minimize this, as does taping the wound for 4–6 weeks following removal of the sutures.

Hypertrophic and keloid scarring. Most people are vulnerable to hypertrophic scarring in the cape area (shoulders and upper trunk), and it tends to complicate wound infection. Some people are particularly susceptible to this type of scarring, which may occur on other areas as well. It is important to ask the patient about the healing from previous surgery and take precautions to minimize this. Precautions include:
- antibiotic prophylaxis for elective procedures
- taking care to avoid wound tension by undermining
- judicious use of deep sutures
- everting the wound edges
- injecting triamcinolone into the wound at the time of suture removal (in some cases).

Taping such wounds postoperatively to splint the skin externally and minimize torsional forces is also important.

When hypertrophic scarring has formed, it can often be improved by intralesional triamcinolone, repeated at 6-weekly intervals as required, and wound splinting with tape, a hydrocolloid dressing or silicon sheeting. Re-excision is best left to experts as the resulting scar may be even worse than the original one.

Koebner phenomenon. Certain skin conditions may localize in scar tissue – psoriasis, lichen planus, warts and even herpes simplex.

Comorbidity

Some medical conditions are associated with surgical complications. These are listed in Table 5.1.

TABLE 5.1

Medical conditions associated with surgical complications

Condition and associated problems	Required treatment
Rheumatic fever/artificial heart valves	
Risk of inducing bacterial endocarditis	Necessitates the use of antibiotic prophylaxis; a broad-spectrum antibiotic in line with local protocol may be required
Joint prosthesis	
Small risk of inducing a septic arthritis or osteomyelitis if the patient becomes septicemic	Consider antibiotic prophylaxis in line with local protocol
Diabetes mellitus	
Potentially poor peripheral circulation	Take great care with extremities
Increased risk of infection	Consider antibiotic prophylaxis
Slower wound healing	Requires close follow-up
Immunocompromised patients	
Increased risk of infection	Consider antibiotic prophylaxis
Slower wound healing	Requires close follow-up
Psoriasis	
Koebner phenomenon	Counsel patient

CONTINUED

TABLE 5.1 (CONTINUED)

Condition and associated problems	Required treatment
Eczema Patients with active dermatitis may be colonized with bacteria, increasing the risk of infection	Consider antibiotic prophylaxis
Peripheral vascular disease Poor circulation leading to slow wound healing and increased risk of infection	Requires close follow-up Consider antibiotic prophylaxis
Rheumatoid arthritis, chronic sun damage, Cushing's disease (including iatrogenic) Paper-thin skin predisposing to wound dehiscence and easy bruising	Awareness of the problem and use of appropriate techniques
Bleeding disorders, e.g. uremia, chronic liver disease, hemophilia, von Willebrand's disease Increased bleeding and hematoma formation	Awareness of the problem; counsel patient
Hypertension Increased bleeding and hematoma formation	Awareness of the problem; counsel patient

Drugs

Some medications increase the risk of complications during or after surgery. Acetylsalicylic acid (aspirin), other non-steroidal anti-inflammatory drugs and anticoagulants are associated with increased bleeding and hematoma formation. Oral and long-term, high-dose inhaled steroids are associated with poor skin quality. Patients taking these drugs, or other immunosuppressants, are potentially immuno-compromised, which may lead to an increased risk of infection and slower wound healing.

Appropriate techniques

Assessment of skin tension lines. Incision along the line of maximum
skin tension will tend to produce the least tension across the wound,
making closure easier and reducing the likelihood of splay scarring in
the longer term. The identification and use of skin tension lines are
discussed in detail in Chapter 4, pages 53–5.

Atraumatic technique. The edges of any wound should be treated as
gently as possible. Crushing of skin by over-vigorous pressure from
instruments will result in inflammation, the possibility of poorly viable
tissue within the wound and damage to the vascular structures involved
in healing. Trauma can be minimized by gentle handling of the edge
using a skin hook or toothed forceps. The use of non-toothed forceps
is best avoided, as the surgeon risks compressing the tissue more firmly
to obtain a grip; even toothed forceps cause crushing as the tissue is
compressed between the jaws. Figure 5.3 shows the correct use of a
skin hook within the wound, which minimizes tissue damage and
promotes healing. Adequate hemostasis is critical; if it is not achieved,
a hematoma may keep the wound edges apart, delay healing and act
as a reservoir for infection.

Sterile technique. Careful attention to sterile technique will minimize
introduction of infection into the wound during surgery. Adequate
hemostasis and avoiding devascularization of the wound edges through
tension will also help prevent infection.

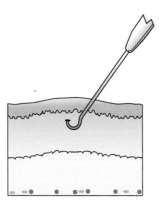

Figure 5.3 Correct use of the
skin hook. The hook is used to
steady the tissue from within the
wound. The overlying skin is
therefore undamaged.

Aftercare

It is important that patients are aware of the factors involved in the aftercare of their wound. Advice can be provided verbally but it may be beneficial to devise a simple patient information leaflet that covers the following items.

Removal of sutures. Sutures will need to be removed from the head and neck in 5–7 days, from the upper limb and trunk at 10 days, and from the lower limbs at 14 days. The longer the sutures remain in the wound, the greater the chance of producing a 'laddered' scar (Figure 5.4) or of the wound becoming infected. Infection of a sutured wound will cause pain and may sometimes cause the wound to dehisce to produce a widened hyperemic scar. If recognized early, infection may be controlled with antibiotics. However, if pus is present within the wound, it may be necessary to remove sutures early to allow free drainage.

Pain. The patient should be aware that the wound might be painful when the local anesthetic wears off, but that any pain should lessen gradually with time. Paracetamol (acetaminophen) is a safer analgesic to administer than aspirin postoperatively, at least in the first 24 hours, to avoid the slight risk of postoperative bleeding. Increasing pain may be a sign of infection or bruising; the patient should be told to seek advice if this occurs.

Bleeding. Simple pressure may be sufficient to control bleeding and the patient should be counseled to press firmly on the wound for 10 minutes. Oozing from the wound edges or from a superficial wound is to be expected; the patient should be advised to seek help if bleeding is persistent or blood loss is great.

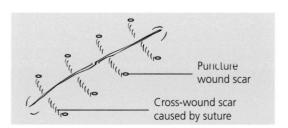

Puncture wound scar

Cross-wound scar caused by suture

Figure 5.4 A laddered scar.

Bruising. Some bruising is inevitable and patients should be warned before surgery that this may occur. Formation of a periorbital hematoma is common following surgery to structures around the eye. Swelling or pain in the area operated on may indicate significant amounts of blood within the wound, which may impede healing. It is wise to ask patients to report any problems so that their situation can be reassessed if necessary. Occasionally, a wound will need to be re-opened to evacuate a clot.

Wound review. The surgeon must decide when to review the wound. Although some surgeons delegate this responsibility to a nurse, there is much to be gained by reviewing your own patients at the time of suture removal. Complex surgery or wounds under tension may require earlier review and dressing changes. Follow-up at an interval, which will depend on local practice and the type of malignancy, is mandatory in skin-cancer surgery. At follow-up, the patient can be examined for both local recurrence and the development of new malignancies.

Key points – avoiding complications

- Surgical logbooks can be used to audit complications so that once a problem has been identified surgical practice can be modified to ensure ongoing improvement.
- Awareness of important underlying structures that run superficially (sometimes only millimeters below the skin surface) will help to avoid damage during skin surgery.
- Infection must be recognized early and appropriate steps taken (e.g. a broad-spectrum antibiotic).
- Any evidence of persistent motor-nerve or tendon damage requires urgent referral to a specialist center.
- Careful attention to technique can minimize trauma to surrounding tissue, introduction of infection and long-term scarring.
- Patients should be made aware of the importance of appropriate aftercare.

There are many different methods of skin closure, not all of which use suture material. Sterile skin-closure strips may be used as an alternative to suture, or after suture removal to strengthen the wound for a few extra days as the healing process matures. Used alone, strips do not evert the wound edges and may lead to a depressed scar. Use of cyanoacrylate glue to close lacerations has gained popularity in emergency departments. However, it cannot be used if there is wound tension (e.g. with an elliptical excision), and it will not evert the wound edges. The cosmetic results may be less favorable than with simple suture.

A practitioner performing excision surgery should master a number of basic suture techniques. These are best practiced on artificial or animal skin (traditionally pigs' trotters) under the supervision of someone experienced in the various techniques. The following descriptions relate to synthetic sutures mounted on a curved reverse-cutting needle using instrument ties (Figure 6.1). Square knots described below are advised to ensure security and prevent slippage with time. Hand tying of knots is an alternative, but this potentially uses more suture material.

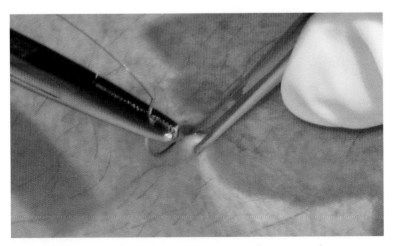

Figure 6.1 Insertion of a synthetic suture mounted on a curved reverse-cutting needle.

The simple interrupted suture

The needle is positioned correctly within the holder, with the middle third of the needle within the jaws (Figure 6.2a). One wound edge is gripped and slightly everted; the needle is pushed into the skin at 90° and, using the curve of the needle, advanced into the center of the wound. The tip should emerge in the subcutaneous fat, or lower dermis on thicker skin, for example on the back (Figure 6.2b). The opposite edge of the wound should be slightly everted and the needle advanced in an equal but opposite action using the curve of the needle (Figure 6.2c). The tip of the needle is retrieved using tissue forceps, not fingers, and the thread is pulled through leaving 2–3 cm at its tail end. The suture is tied using a square knot.

- The initial 'throw' of the suture is double, and is pulled firmly but not tightly. The second throw is single and should be opposite to the initial one, forming a reef knot, which is stable. (If the first throw is anticlockwise around the needle holder, then the second should be clockwise.)

- The longer end of the suture, with the needle on, is twisted twice around the suture holder in an anticlockwise fashion. (Move the needle holder rather than the suture as this minimizes the risk from the needle.) The needle holder then grips the short end of the suture. The first throw of the knot is tied by pulling one end of the suture at 180° to the other, usually across the wound. This should appose the wound edges (Figure 6.2d).

- The second (or locking) throw of the suture is made by twisting the thread once in a clockwise direction around the holder and pulling closed as before. It is this throw that determines the tension within the completed suture. The operator should ensure that, though tight enough to appose the wound, this throw is not so tight as to cause tissue bunching or even an ischemic area (Figure 6.2e).

- The third throw is anticlockwise and single. The final knot should be pulled to one side of the wound and not allowed to overlie the wound edges, as this leads to chafing and may allow infection into the completed wound (Figure 6.2f).

- The final track of the suture within the skin is shown in Figure 6.2g. Interrupted sutures should be spaced evenly, and should draw the

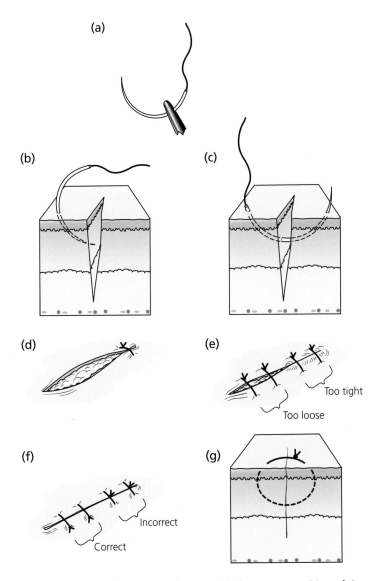

Figure 6.2 The simple interrupted suture. (a) The correct position of the needle in the needle holder. (b, c) The desired path of the suture through the skin. (d) Apposition of the wound edge is achieved by the first double throw of the knot. (e) After the second throw of the knot, the tension should be adjusted. (f) Knots should not lie directly over the wound. (g) The final track of the suture within the skin.

wound together without leaving redundant tissue at either end of the wound (a dog-ear). This may be achieved either by marking the ellipse with cross-reference points (see Figure 4.2c, page 53) or by the technique of 'halving', in which the first suture is placed at the center point of the wound and the resulting deficits progressively halved until the desired effect is achieved (Figure 6.3).

The vertical mattress suture

This is an alternative to the simple interrupted suture in wounds that are under tension. It is not a substitute for buried intradermal sutures, but may be used in areas where the dermis is too friable to hold a buried suture. A combination of vertical mattress and simple interrupted sutures may be used.

The skin is punctured twice on each side of the wound. A deep, wide 'bite' is taken first, then a smaller reverse bite is taken in the same plane. A square knot is then tied as before (Figure 6.4).

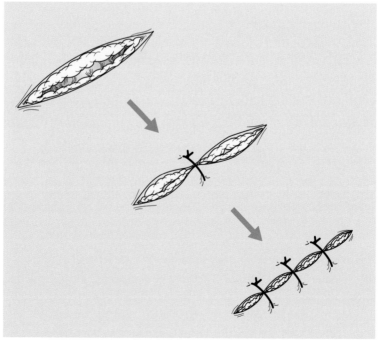

Figure 6.3 The 'halving' technique.

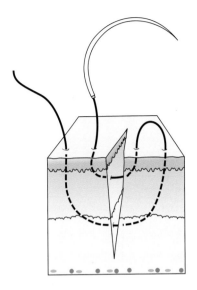

Figure 6.4 The vertical mattress suture.

The buried intradermal suture

This is used to remove the tension from wound edges. Absorbable suture material is used that retains its tensile strength for a number of weeks as the wound matures. Using a 3-0 or 4-0 absorbable suture, such as Vicryl®, one edge of the wound is everted, and, starting from deep within the wound, a bite of tissue including the dermis is taken (Figure 6.5a). The opposite edge is everted, and an equal bite is taken superficially and ending deep (Figure 6.5b).

Care must be taken to line up opposite sides of the wound. The two edges are pulled together, taking the tension off the surface of the skin, the suture is tied with a square knot and the ends cut short. The knot is buried in the wound and the wound edges should now approximate with little or no tension (Figure 6.5c). (A larger wound may need three or four buried sutures.)

The running or continuous suture

This is useful in apposing wound edges that are under little tension or after insertion of buried intradermal sutures. It has the advantage of being quick and easy to insert, and apposes the wound edges well. It may be 'locked' to hold the edges together more effectively, but this causes greater suture marks.

75

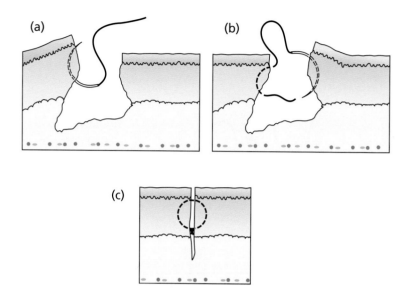

Figure 6.5 The buried intradermal suture. (a) Starting from deep within the wound a bite of tissue including dermis is taken. (b) The opposite edge is everted and an equal bite is taken superficially and ending deep. (c) The knot is buried in the wound.

A simple skin suture is inserted in one end of the wound and repeated loops are made through the skin. The suture is pulled until the edges appose, but is not pulled tight, to allow for tissue swelling after surgery (Figure 6.6a). The end is tied to the final loop. To lock the running suture, the needle, as it emerges from the skin, is hooked under the previous loop (Figure 6.6b).

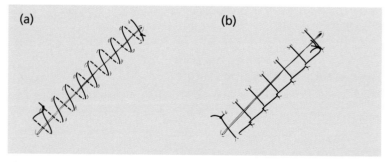

Figure 6.6 (a) The simple running suture. (b) The locked running suture.

The running subcuticular suture

This is a dermal suture that removes the risk of suture marks. It may remain in place for longer than simple interrupted sutures and can be valuable in areas that are likely to heal poorly. Monofilament non-absorbable sutures should be used because other materials will absorb fluid and swell. The suture must be sufficiently strong to withstand the force needed to pull it through the skin at removal; 4-0 Prolene® is ideal.

The needle is introduced approximately 3 mm away from the tip of the wound and advanced into the center of the incision. A small bite is taken in the dermis on one side of the wound, with the needle held in the same plane as the skin surface. An equal but opposite bite is taken from the other edge slightly further down the wound. In this way, the suture is advanced down the length of the wound 3–5 mm at a time (Figure 6.7a). When the far end of the wound is reached, the needle is advanced from the center of the wound to the skin surface some 3 mm outside the wound. Both ends of the suture are gripped and pulled gently, so that the wound edges appose. Both ends may be taped to the skin using adhesive wound closures or the ends may be tied back on themselves with knots (Figure 6.7b).

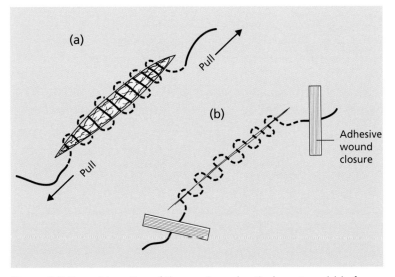

Figure 6.7 Correct insertion of the running subcuticular suture: (a) before and (b) after the application of tension to close the deficit.

The tip suture

Occasionally, a corner or tip of a piece of skin may need to be sutured into a defect. The tip may have a compromised blood supply and insertion of simple sutures may threaten tissue viability. In this case, a half-buried horizontal mattress suture should be used.

The needle is inserted into the skin 3 mm away from the deficit into which the tip is to be sutured and emerges into the deficit in the deep dermis. Within the deep dermis, the needle then picks up the tip and finally passes out of the deficit through the deep dermis and emerges 3 mm away from the deficit (Figure 6.8). It is important that the part of the suture above the skin does not overlie the tip as this may reduce tissue viability.

The leveling suture

If an ellipse of skin has been removed, the wound edges to be apposed may differ in thickness (Figure 6.9a), for example near the eye. It is important for cosmetics that the edges are apposed accurately, which can be achieved using a leveling suture.

Various techniques can be used to achieve the desired effect. A modified simple suture may be used where the bite taken out of the higher or thicker skin surface is less than the bite taken from the lower or thinner one (Figure 6.9b). A similar modification may be made to the inverted mattress suture to achieve leveling (Figure 6.9c).

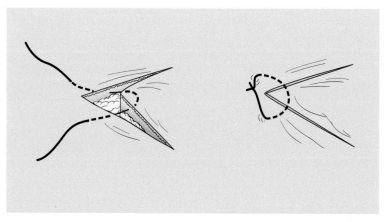

Figure 6.8 The tip suture.

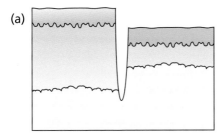

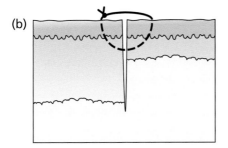

Figure 6.9 (a) Wound edges with differing skin thickness/levels. (b) A simple interrupted leveling suture. (c) A vertical mattress leveling suture.

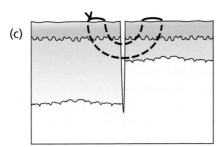

'Tying off' for hemostasis

Tying off blood vessels is an alternative to cautery for hemostasis and is the best method to control bleeding from arterioles and larger veins. It is the only method that should be used in larger arterial systems, such as the temple, as cauterized vessels in this area may bleed shortly after the operation, leading to hematoma formation.

The offending vessel is identified and, using artery forceps (hemostat), the cut end is clipped to control bleeding. The simplest solution is to tie a simple suture directly around the vessel, but larger vessels should be attached to surrounding tissue to ensure the security of the suture (Figure 6.10).

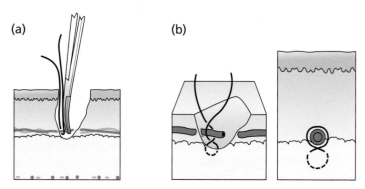

Figure 6.10 Tying off blood vessels. (a) A simple tie is eased over the tip of an artery forceps (hemostat). (b) Anchoring a blood vessel to surrounding tissue for stability.

Suture removal

The removal technique depends on the type of suture. Always ensure that the person removing the sutures is familiar with the techniques involved. When removing sutures, it is important not to exert vertical pressure on the wound, and not to pull material that has been on the surface, and is therefore potentially infected, through the wound.

Simple interrupted sutures should be removed using sharp, thin-bladed scissors. The suture is cut as closely to the skin surface as possible and, with gentle traction at 90° to the wound edge, the suture is removed parallel to the skin surface (Figure 6.11a).

Vertical mattress sutures should be cut next to the knot near the skin surface. The deep loop is then pulled through and cut near the skin surface on the opposite side of the wound. The remaining superficial loop may be removed by traction on the knot (Figure 6.11b).

Continuous or running sutures should be removed in small sections to minimize wound contamination (Figure 6.11c).

A continuous subcuticular suture is removed by trimming one end as it emerges from the skin and pulling on the other end, while applying gentle counter-traction on the wound (Figure 6.11d). If it is not possible

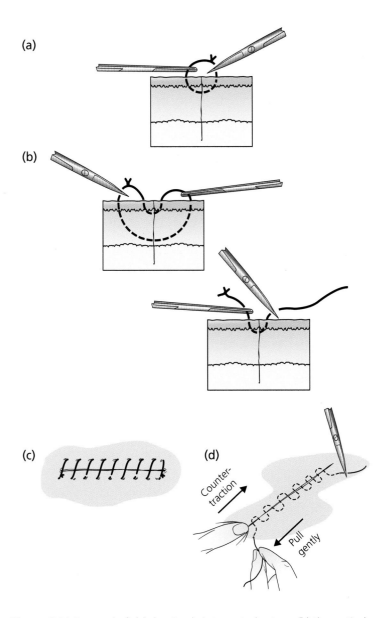

Figure 6.11 Removal of. (a) the simple interrupted suture; (b) the vertical mattress suture in two stages; (c) the continuous or running suture in short sections to minimize wound contamination; (d) the running subcuticular suture by gentle traction.

to pull the subcuticular suture through completely, it should be cut as short as possible and the end allowed to retract back into the wound. Modern monofilament sutures are well tolerated and will eventually reabsorb.

Key points – suturing techniques and removal

- Suturing is best practiced on artificial or animal skin under the supervision of someone experienced in the various techniques.
- Square knots are advised, to ensure security and prevent slippage with time; hand tying of knots is an alternative but uses more suture material.
- Buried intradermal sutures are used to remove the tension from wound edges.
- Vertical mattress sutures may be suitable for wounds that are under tension, where the dermis is too friable to hold a buried suture.
- Running subcuticular sutures can be left in place for longer than simple interrupted sutures and are therefore valuable in areas of poor healing.
- Tying off blood vessels is the best method to control bleeding from arterioles and larger veins, and is the only method that should be used in larger arterial systems.
- Vertical pressure should not be exerted on the wound during suture removal, and material that has been on the surface should not be pulled through the wound.

Proper use of the correct surgical technique for the diagnosis is the basis of successful minor surgery. Cutting lesions off patients is easy; the difficulty arises in repairing the damage you have done. Good pre-operative diagnosis, treatment planning and use of the most appropriate and minimally invasive methods will optimize your surgical results.

Snip excision

This is appropriate for skin tags or narrow-necked fibro-epithelial polyps. The lesion is anesthetized if necessary but often the injection of anesthetic is more painful than the snip. The growth is then held firmly in a pair of tissue forceps and the neck of the tag or polyp is cut with sharp scissors (Figure 7.1). To control bleeding, chemical solutions (e.g. aluminum hydrochloride) may be applied to the base of the lesion or it may be heat cauterized; however, pressure is usually sufficient.

Cautery excision

This procedure is again appropriate for skin tags, but also for wider-necked fibro-epithelial polyps. Local anesthesia is normally used; instead of using scissors, the neck is divided using a cutting cautery tip; hemostasis is usually instant (Figure 7.2).

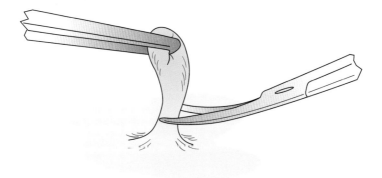

Figure 7.1 Snip excision.

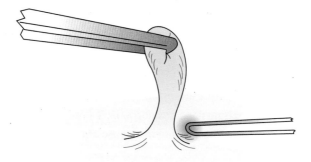

Figure 7.2 Cautery excision.

Shave excision

This technique is appropriate for raised benign lesions (Figure 7.3). The lesion is anesthetized by raising it on a mound of anesthetic; a large scalpel blade or surgical razor is used to shave the lesion off its 'mound' using a fine sawing action (Figure 7.4). Pressure is often sufficient for hemostasis. Alternatively, hemostatic solutions (e.g. aluminum hydrochloride) can be used. Heat cautery may exaggerate the scarring and should be avoided if possible.

Shave biopsy. The shave excision technique may be used to biopsy suspected basal cell carcinoma (BCC) or squamous cell carcinoma (SCC), but is not appropriate for biopsy of suspected malignant melanomas as the histological thickness of the lesion is used to plan definitive surgery and determine the prognosis.

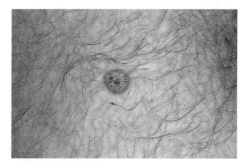

Figure 7.3 A lesion suitable for shave excision.

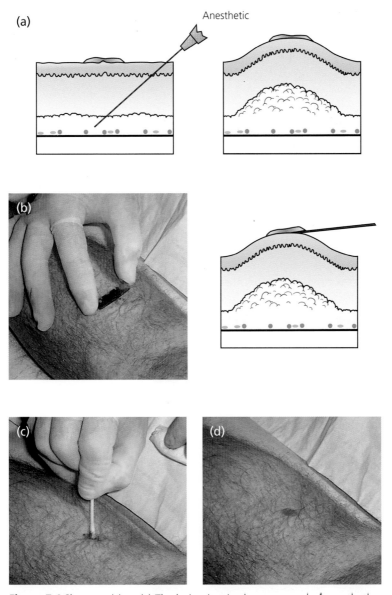

Figure 7.4 Shave excision. (a) The lesion is raised on a mound of anesthetic.
(b) A large surgical razor is used to shave the lesion off its mound.
(c) A hemostatic solution of aluminum hydrochloride is applied on a cotton
bud. d) The outcome of shave excision.

85

Punch biopsy

This procedure is appropriate for diagnosis of many lesions, such as actinic (solar) keratoses, Bowen's disease, BCC or SCC. However, it may not be appropriate for biopsy of pigmented lesions. A 3-mm biopsy is usually sufficient for diagnosis of a lesion, but a larger biopsy may be required for diagnosis of a rash, such as granuloma annulare.

The lesion is marked and anesthetized. The skin punch is then pressed with a firm twisting action onto an active part of the lesion. The core is carefully raised with toothed forceps or a skin hook to avoid crushing the tissue and, if required, the neck is snipped with scissors (Figure 7.5).

When a 2–4-mm punch is used, the wound does not usually require suture or cautery, except on the scalp, where, unless pressure can be applied for 10–15 minutes, a suture is advisable. The deficit from a 6-mm punch (or 4-mm punch taken in a cosmetically sensitive area) will benefit from a small suture. In this case, the skin should be stretched when taking the punch so that the resultant defect is oval rather than round (Figure 7.6). This allows better approximation of the wound and avoids dog-ears. Great care should be taken if this technique is used on the nose as it may result in a depressed and noticeable scar.

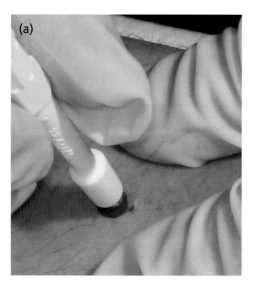

(a)

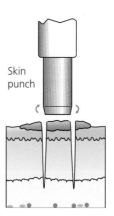

Skin punch

Figure 7.5 Punch biopsy. (a) The skin punch is pressed with a firm, twisting action onto an active area of the lesion.

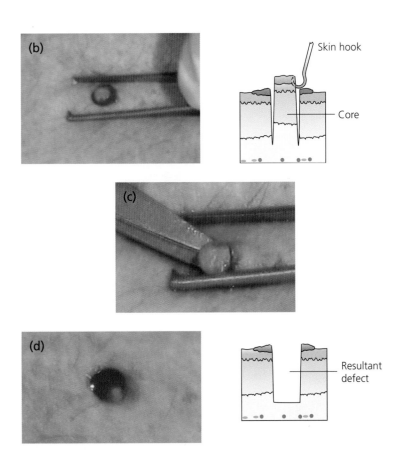

Figure 7.5 Punch biopsy *(CONTINUED)*. (b) The core is raised with a skin hook or toothed forceps. (c) If necessary, the neck is snipped with scissors. (d) The resultant defect does not usually require suturing.

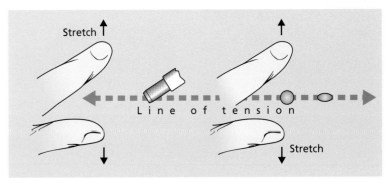

Figure 7.6 Producing an oval deficit that is easier to close.

Curettage

This is the most appropriate surgical intervention for viral warts and seborrheic keratoses. The lesion is anesthetized and, using a sharp Volkmann or disposable curette, the lesion is literally scraped off the skin (Figure 7.7) while the skin is held taut with the other hand. This will rarely cause more than oozing of blood from the surface of a

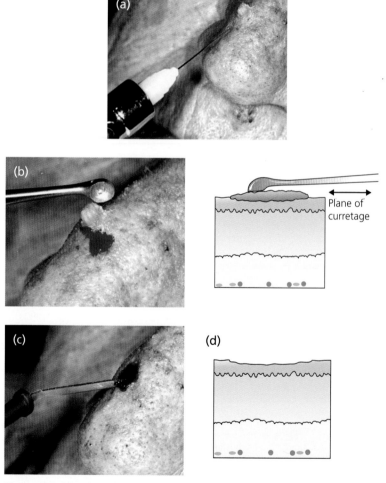

Figure 7.7 Curettage. (a) The lesion is anesthetized. (b) The lesion is scraped off with a curette. (c) Coagulation is achieved, if necessary, using electrodesiccation. (d) The outcome of curettage is minimal dermal insult.

seborrheic keratosis, which can be dealt with easily by pressure, aluminum chloride, light cautery or electrodesiccation.

A pyogenic granuloma is a vascular tumor and will respond well to curettage; however, cautery of the central feeder vessel will be required. The main practical point is to limit the insult to the dermis; the plane of curettage should therefore be parallel to the skin surface. This is particularly important when using a disposable curette as deep furrows may be cut with its sharp surgical blade.

Incisional biopsy

It is sometimes appropriate to take a biopsy from a lesion by incising part of it. This technique gives a larger and deeper sample than punch biopsy, and is particularly useful in the diagnosis of paniculitis (e.g. erythema nodosum) and morphea, where some normal perilesional skin is required. It is also useful for debulking a large patch of Bowen's disease or a BCC.

Initially, part of the lesion is removed for biopsy; the remainder is removed surgically at a later date (Figure 7.8). Although two procedures are necessary, it may save a single, larger intervention such as a skin graft, and the resultant scar is shorter.

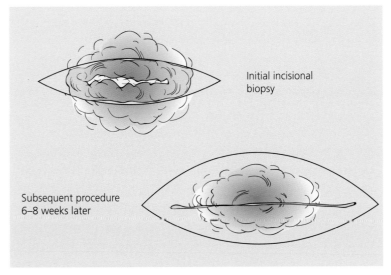

Initial incisional biopsy

Subsequent procedure 6–8 weeks later

Figure 7.8 Incisional biopsy and two-stage procedure.

89

Excision (biopsy)

This is appropriate for 'suspicious' (suspect) pigmented lesions, keratoacanthomas, Bowen's disease, SCC and BCC. It should be reserved for lesions for which the surgeon has made a confident diagnosis and for which excision is the treatment of choice. It is important to remember that it is easier to excise a BCC completely first time than to do so at a subsequent session. The surgeon should be confident in techniques of wound closure before opening a wound. Suture techniques should be practiced under supervision and a variety of techniques should be at the surgeon's disposal (Table 7.1).

There is a structured procedure for excision.

- *Identify and mark the lesion with an appropriate excision margin* (Figure 7.9a). Plan the orientation of the incision, taking into account skin tension lines (see Figure 4.3, page 54), surrounding structures and the long axis of the lesion. Mark the ellipse with a 2.5–3:1 ratio (Figure 7.9b).
- *Anesthetize the area.*
- *Incise both edges.* Using a No. 15 blade, starting at the tip and with the skin under tension, make an incision following the outside edge of the skin marking (Figure 7.9c). The point of the wound should be made with the blade at 90° to the skin. The incision should be smooth and sure so that one side of the ellipse is incised using a single sweep of the blade. At the end of the sweep, ensure that the blade is again at 90° to the skin and that the incision does not cross the mid-line of the marked ellipse at the tip. The procedure is then repeated on the other half of the ellipse. Cross-ends should be avoided, as should multiple 'slashes' on the incision borders (Figure 7.9d).
- *Deepen the wound.* The area of skin should now be made into an 'island' by following the line of the incision with sharp dissecting scissors, cutting at 90° to the skin surface. This should then leave an area of skin on a fatty island (Figure 7.9e).
- *Remove the lesion.* The lesion can then be removed quickly and cleanly by holding the apex of the ellipse with a skin hook (or toothed forceps) and cutting through the subcuticular fat with a pair of sharp dissecting scissors. This should leave a wound with sides that are perpendicular to the surface, down to a flat base (Figure 7.9f).

TABLE 7.1

Knowledge and skills potentially required for excision surgery

Lesion recognition and planning

- Excision surgery to be used for a limited range of lesions; planning of closure, particularly with reference to surrounding structures

Regional anatomy

- Knowledge of the location of important nerves and blood vessels that run superficially (see Chapter 5, pages 60–4)

Correct manipulation of full range of instruments

- Correct use of instruments to improve operative technique and reduce trauma to surrounding skin

Sterile technique

- To reduce the risk of infection

Excision technique

- To fully excise the lesion and to leave a wound that closes with minimal effort

Undermining

- Important when the skin is under tension

Hemostatic techniques

- Familiarity with manipulation of artery forceps, the use of the cautery machine and techniques of tying off blood vessels to stop bleeding within a wound

Buried dermal suture

- To take the tension out of all but the smallest of wounds

Skin suturing

- Knowledge of several suturing methods to close the wound; a reasonable range may include interrupted simple skin sutures, running intradermal sutures and vertical mattress sutures

Dog-ear repair

- To prevent scarring that is likely to be cosmetically poor

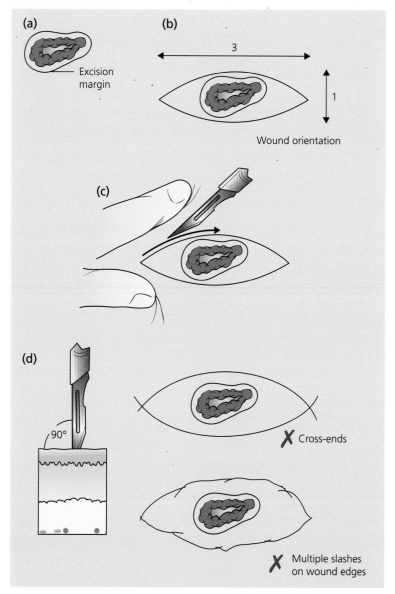

Figure 7.9 Excision. (a, b) Marking a lesion. (c) Tension is applied to the skin and the initial incision is made, starting and finishing the sweep with the blade at 90°, (d) avoiding cross-ends and multiple slashes. (e) The wound is deepened to the fat layer. (f) The lesion is removed to leave a wound with sides perpendicular to a flat base. (g) Undermining in the plane of the base.

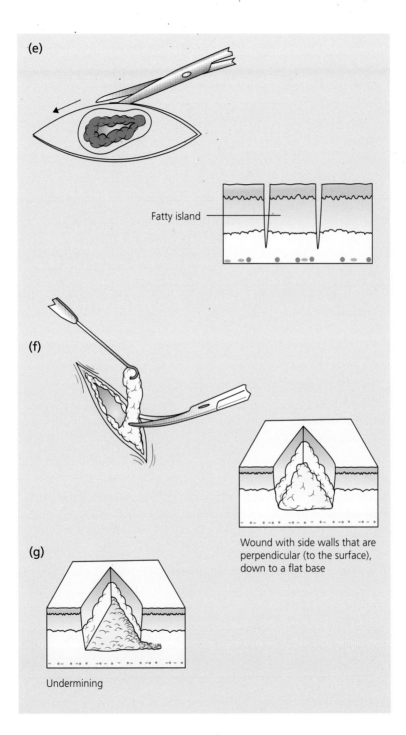

(e)

Fatty island

(f)

Wound with side walls that are perpendicular (to the surface), down to a flat base

(g)

Undermining

- *Undermine*, i.e. separate the dermis from the underlying fat layer using dissecting scissors (Figure 7.9g). Undermining allows the edges of the wound to be pulled together over the deficit more easily so that the wound is under less tension. The extent to which undermining is necessary depends on the width of the wound and the tension of the surrounding skin. The wider the wound and the tighter the skin, the greater the need for undermining.
- *Hemostasis* should be achieved before insertion of sutures.
- *Buried dermal sutures*. If any tension remains on the skin, buried interrupted dermal sutures should be inserted (see pages 75–6). These should be used in all but the smallest (1–2 cm) excisions.
- *Skin sutures*. The choice of suture used to close the skin depends on the site of the wound. For the face and neck, 6-0 or 5-0 monofilament (e.g. Ethilon®) should be used; 4-0 or 3-0 monofilament may be appropriate elsewhere. Interrupted skin sutures are inserted, taking small equal bites either side of the wound and making sure that the edges are approximated (see pages 72–3). It is important that the edges are slightly everted to avoid a depressed scar. Sutures should be inserted alternately at either end of the wound and equidistant.

Dog-ear repair

Occasionally, when repairing a wound, a flap of redundant skin called a dog-ear will loop up at one end or in the center due to uneven apposition of the wound edges (Figure 7.10a). This may be as a result of inaccurate apposition of the wound edges or because skin tension pulls the wound at an oblique angle.

Cross-marking the wound before incision, or applying tension to each end of the wound with skin hooks, may avoid dog-ears because this allows easier and more accurate apposition of the wound (Figure 7.10b).

The extra skin should be excised; if left, it will heal, leaving a proud area. The excess fold is tented with a skin hook and laid over to one side (Figure 7.10c). Using a scalpel, the base of the triangle thus formed is incised, the fold is then laid over to the other side and another incision is made. The two incisions should meet at the apex and the triangle of skin is removed (Figure 7.10d). The resulting defect should be closed using interrupted sutures (Figure 7.10e).

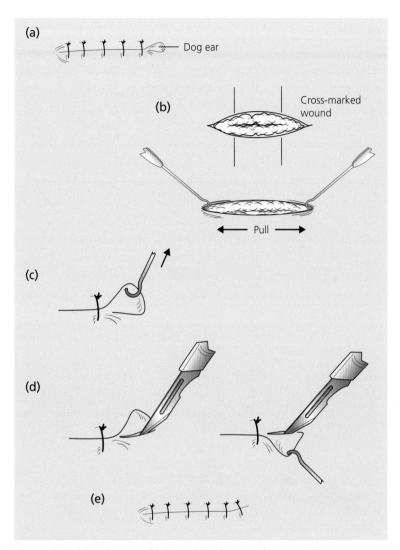

Figure 7.10 (a) A dog-ear. (b) To avoid a dog-ear, the wound is cross-marked before incision, or tension is applied to each end of the wound with skin hooks. (c) To repair a dog-ear, the excess fold is tented with a skin hook and laid over to one side. (d) Using a scalpel, the base of the triangle thus formed is incised, the fold is then laid over to the other side and another incision is made. The two incisions should meet at the apex and the triangle of skin is removed. (e) The resulting defect is closed using interrupted sutures.

95

Partial closure

When dealing with a large wound under tension or in an area close to facial features, it is sometimes preferable to partially close the wound to reduce the tension and avoid deforming adjacent structures.

The wound is made and, using a variety of techniques including generous undermining and tension sutures, the skin is mobilized to its maximum extent. In this case, closure is best performed from the ends towards the center. Once tension or distortion is evident, the central defect is left to heal by secondary intention (Figure 7.11a). The central defect may be held closer using sterile skin strips. The risk of infection in this type of wound is greater than in a closed wound and the use of prophylactic antibiotics should be considered. The resultant scar will be widened in the central unsutured area, but this is preferable to distortion of features. A variation on this is partial closure of a wound leaving a defect at one end; this is useful beneath the eye (Figures 7.11b, c).

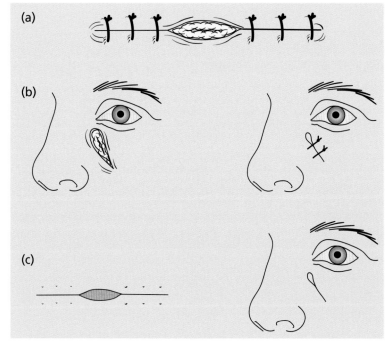

Figure 7.11 (a) Partial closure to leave a central defect. (b) Partial closure of a wound beneath the eye leaving a defect at one end. (c) The resultant scars.

Chondrodermatitis nodularis chronica helicis

The pathological process involved in this lesion is limited to the cartilage underlying the inflamed skin. The nodule within the cartilage is identified and marked. Local anesthetic is infiltrated around the area. Because the ear is supplied by end arteries, in theory lidocaine without epinephrine (adrenaline) should be used. The ear is, however, well supplied with vessels and in practice epinephrine can be used in many patients, with the exception of those with signs of poor perfusion or possibly diabetes mellitus.

When the anesthetic has taken effect, a straight incision or small ellipse is made and the overlying skin is reflected back, exposing the cartilage. The nodule is excised and, most importantly, the surrounding area of cartilage is pared down flat (Figure 7.12). The skin is then closed over the deficit. The problem may recur, particularly if the nodule is not fully excised or if sharp edges are left on the cartilage.

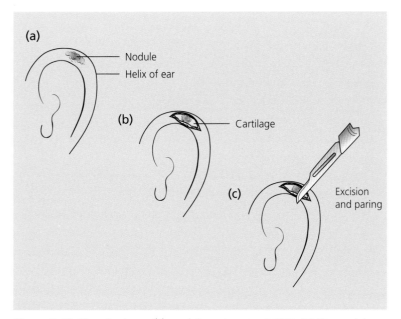

Figure 7.12 Chondrodermatitis nodularis chronica helicis. (a) The nodule within the cartilage is identified and marked. (b) The overlying skin is reflected back, exposing the cartilage. (c) The nodule is excised and the surrounding area of cartilage is pared down flat.

97

Epidermoid cysts

Epidermoid cysts may arise from epidermis that has implanted and proliferated in the subcutaneous tissue or dermis, or may represent occlusion of a pilo-sebaceous follicle. They are common on the head and neck and also occur on the trunk and limbs.

An epidermal cyst appears as a slowly enlarging spherical nodule, often with an identifiable punctum connecting to the cyst cavity. A cheesy, white, keratinous discharge may exude through the punctum if the lesion is squeezed.

Epidermoid cysts require surgery if they are large and unsightly or if they have repeatedly become infected, inflamed or have discharged. Surgery should not be undertaken within 4–6 weeks of acute infection as the resultant scar tissue makes surgery difficult.

There is a clear procedure for cyst removal (Figure 7.13).

- *Identify the cyst and mark the incision.* A thin ellipse of skin is excised, including the punctum. The width of the ellipse depends on the size of the cyst. If an ellipse is not excised, then closure will result in spare skin and potentially a space (Figure 7.13a).
- *Anesthetize the area*, taking care not to puncture the cyst. Consider using a field block (see pages 24–5).
- *Make the incision along the lines of maximum skin tension.* Using blunt dissection, with either artery forceps or round-ended curved scissors, attempt to free the cyst from the surrounding tissue. Repeat on all sides of the cyst (Figure 7.13b).
- *Gently lift the cyst* using toothed forceps on the excised skin; use curved scissors to free the base (Figure 7.13c). Cysts often fragment and it is important to excise fragments from the base of the wound in order to minimize the risk of recurrence.
- *Insert a subcuticular or fat stitch* to close the potential space if the cyst was particularly large. Close the skin using interrupted sutures.

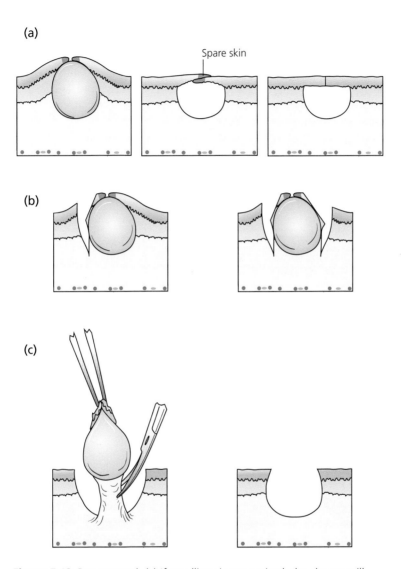

Figure 7.13 Cyst removal. (a) If an ellipse is not excised, the closure will result in spare skin and potentially a space. (b) Blunt dissection to free the cyst. (c) The cyst is removed leaving a deficit.

Abscesses

An abscess is a collection of pus under the skin, which may occur anywhere but is more common in the axilla, groin or perianal region. An axillary or perianal abscess should not be incised in primary care as the extent of the abscess cavity cannot always be judged clinically because of the large amount of loose tissue in these areas.

The treatment of choice is to incise and de-roof the abscess and allow healing by secondary intention (Figure 7.14). It is not appropriate to suture the wound. Any dead tissue overlying the abscess should be trimmed to aid healing. A cruciate incision is sometimes used as this allows access to the deeper areas of the abscess cavity and allows the surgeon to identify any locules of pus within it. A large abscess will require packing with either absorbable or cotton ribbon gauze to allow healing from the base.

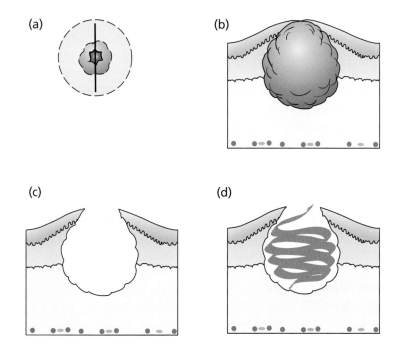

(a)   (b)

(c)   (d)

Figure 7.14 Abscess treatment. (a) The incision is planned to allow free drainage. (b) Pus is sometimes loculated. (c) Pus is expressed leaving a cavity. (d) Packing may be required.

Lipomas

These are often larger than they appear on the surface and surgeons must be prepared for this possibility. Occasionally there may also be vigorous bleeding in the base of the wound.

It is useful to use a skin-marking pen to delineate the borders of a lipoma before infiltrating the area with anesthetic, as the swelling of the infiltrated tissue may obscure the lipoma. Large lipomas can usually be removed through small skin incisions. As the tumor is deep to the skin, it is rarely necessary to remove an ellipse of skin and a straight incision is preferable. The lipoma can often be squeezed out through the incision with massage (Figure 7.15a), negating the need for soft tissue dissection and reducing the risk of bleeding from the base. Occasionally, the lipoma will need to be dissected out around its circumference (Figure 7.14b). Some lipomas have large arterioles running into the

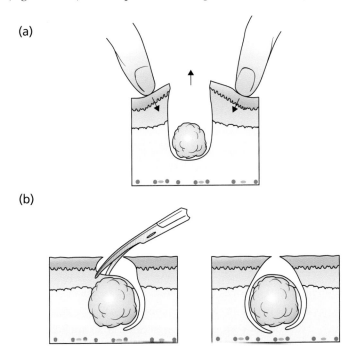

(a)

(b)

Figure 7.15 (a) A lipoma can often be squeezed out through the incision. (b) Occasionally, the lipoma will need to be dissected out around its circumference.

101

base, which may require either cautery or 'tying off'. For larger lipomas, a fat stitch will be required to close the potential space. The skin is closed with interrupted sutures.

Cryosurgery

This technique involves the destruction of tissue by application of a very cold substance. The usual cryogen is liquid nitrogen. The principal aim is to produce an ice ball that can be maintained for a measured length of time that corresponds to the amount of tissue damage required to destroy the lesion. Inflammation is a byproduct of tissue destruction and also contributes to eradication of the lesion. The degree of inflammation is dose-related, but some patients may experience a marked inflammatory reaction with blister formation and erosions.

The process is painful and extreme care is required when using cryosurgery in children. Most children will not tolerate the pain, which limits its use to single warts or the occasional molluscum contagiosum (see page 42). Alternative treatments, such as wart paints, plasters or duct tape, will be required for this group.

There are various ways to apply liquid nitrogen (Table 7.2), but if it is used frequently it is a good idea to invest in a cryoflask with either a spray or probe to direct the treatment. It is also good practice to supply the patient with a written advice sheet after cryosurgery (Figure 7.16).

Applications

Viral warts. Before using cryosurgery, remember that up to 80% of viral warts respond to treatment with paints, gels or duct tape. Also, cryosurgery is painful and most require multiple treatments, usually at 3-weekly intervals. Cryosurgery has a low success rate for plantar warts, which can be extremely painful to treat. In addition, most viral warts are self-limiting over 1–2 years, so reassurance may be the best option.

Actinic (solar) keratoses are benign lesions and may be treated with a cryospray, cryoprobe or cotton-tipped applicator. If an applicator is used, it should be dipped into a foam cup containing decanted liquid nitrogen and then applied directly to the lesion with moderate pressure for 10–15 seconds. An ice ball should be seen to form around the lesion. Home-made, open-weave, cotton-tipped applicators are best, as

TABLE 7.2

Advantages and disadvantages of different cryotherapy methods

Type of applicator	Advantages	Disadvantages
Flask and cotton-wool balls	• Cheap	• No directable spray • Health and safety risk • Potential transport problem
Cryospray	• Directable spray • Range of nozzles available • May also be fitted with cryoprobe	• Expensive initial purchase
Cryoprobe	• No spray, but may be converted to cryospray	• Expensive initial purchase

Patient advice: cryosurgery

You have just received treatment by cryosurgery. This involves an application of liquid nitrogen to freeze and destroy the unhealthy tissue. The area then heals with a growth of healthy new skin.

The treatment is painful; however, the pain subsides within 30–60 seconds. You may notice a throbbing sensation as the skin thaws out. Over the next 2–3 hours, the skin may become red and swollen. Occasionally a blister will form; this is also normal. The blister may be punctured using a needle that has been sterilized in a flame. Later a scab forms over the treated area, which will be shed over the next 5–10 days.

If you have any worries about your treatment please speak to .... on telephone number .... who will be glad to advise you.

Figure 7.16 An advice sheet for cryosurgery patients.

103

proprietary ones retain less liquid nitrogen and consequently require multiple re-dips. Adherence to local health and safety guidelines on the storage and use of liquid nitrogen is mandatory.

Freeze times. The most useful predictors of cure are the freeze time and the number of freeze–thaw cycles applied to a lesion (Table 7.3). Freezing a lesion, allowing it to thaw completely and then refreezing it a second time inflicts substantially greater tissue damage than simply prolonging the freeze time.

Contraindications. Cryosurgery is contraindicated for undiagnosed lesions, particularly undiagnosed pigmented lesions. Also, it should not be used if there is a risk of damage to local structures, such as the eye, underlying tendons, nerves or blood vessels, or on large areas in regions of poorly healing tissue, such as the anterior shin. It may not be suitable for people with Raynaud's phenomenon or cold intolerance.

TABLE 7.3

Freeze times for various lesions

Lesion	Ice-ball time (seconds)	Number of freeze–thaw cycles
Viral warts		
Small	5–10	1 or 2
Large	10–20	1 or 2
Plantar	15–30	2
Solar keratoses		
Thin	10	1 or 2
Thick	15	2
Seborrheic keratoses		
Thin	5–10	1
Thick	15–25	1

Great caution needs to be exercised when using cryosurgery to treat skin malignancy. Careful lesion selection is required. The treatment is suitable for superficial BCCs on the trunk, but is contraindicated for morpheic or recurrent BCCs, or lesions in high-risk sites. In addition, audits have shown that treatment will reliably fail unless two 30-second freeze–thaw cycles are applied, and this is associated with substantial morbidity. Successful cryotherapy of skin cancer therefore requires considerable experience in both diagnosis and practical application.

Toenail surgery

Ingrowing toenails are painful because of chronic inflammation and infection of the lateral margin of the great toenail folds (Figure 7.17). The pathology is restricted to the lateral few millimeters of the nail. Occasionally, other nails become involved, particularly in patients receiving oral retinoids for acne or psoriasis. Predisposing factors include malalignment of the toenails, trauma to the toenails and trimming the nails too short at the corners.

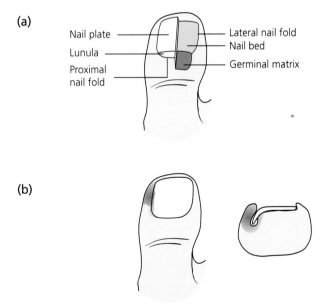

(a)

Nail plate — Lateral nail fold — Nail bed

Lunula —

Proximal nail fold — Germinal matrix

(b)

Figure 7.17 (a) Anatomy of the toenail. (b) Inflammation in the lateral nail fold.

Conservative treatment. In the absence of an underlying nail distortion, surgery is rarely required and the majority of patients can be managed conservatively. This is particularly the case if the lateral incurving is mild or symptoms are new. Elevation of the lateral border of the nail with a cotton-wool plug over the inflamed skin, and allowing the nail to grow distally beyond the nail bed, usually remedies the situation (Figure 7.18a). Advising patients to cut the nail 'square' to the tip of the toe will help to prevent relapse. Review at 6 weeks, as other interventions may be required if this is not successful.

Other conservative measures include grooving the nail with a file or cutting a V-shaped deficit in the center of the nail in an effort to reduce the pressure in the lateral nail folds (Figure 7.18b). However, these measures have a low success rate.

Trimming the nail within the fold is painful and repeated treatments are required (Figure 7.18c). This will give temporary relief from pain and allows drainage of necrotic material and pus. The resolution of the inflammation is sometimes sufficient to allow more normal positioning of nail regrowth; good nail hygiene may then be sufficient to avoid recurrence.

Surgery. Toenail surgery in primary care should be avoided in patients with diabetes, peripheral vascular disease and neuropathy. Methods include:
- avulsion
- lateral avulsion with phenolization of the lateral nail matrix
- nail matrix surgery.

Avulsion. Simple avulsion of the nail allows time for the inflammation in the fold to subside. Regrowth may be normal in up to 50% of cases. However, if the condition is chronic or the anatomy of the nail is altered, simple avulsion is not the treatment of choice. Similarly, recurrence after simple avulsions indicates that repeat avulsion will probably have the same outcome. Alternative therapies such as lateral avulsion with phenolization of the lateral nail matrix should be considered in such cases.

In avulsion, the toe is anesthetized using a ring block and the operative field should then be checked for sensation. The toe is

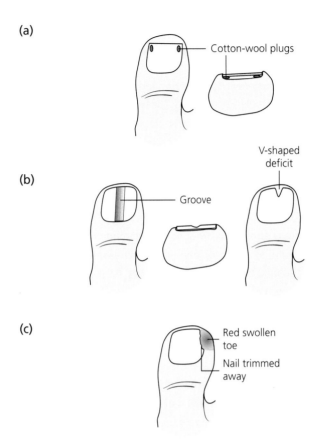

Figure 7.18 Conservative treatment of an ingrowing toenail. (a) Cotton-wool plugs are used to elevate the lateral aspect of the nail. (b) A V-shaped cut or groove may be made in the center of the nail to reduce the pressure in the lateral nail folds. (c) Trimming the nail within the fold.

exsanguinated and a tourniquet applied. The nail is then separated carefully from the nail bed and avulsed using strong artery forceps with a twisting pulling action. Excess granulation tissue is excised or curetted from the nail fold. Next, the tourniquet is removed and pressure applied to the nail bed for 2 minutes. The toe is then dressed with a non-adherent dressing, such as paraffin gauze, or iodine if infection is present.

Postoperative care includes simple analgesia, wearing open-toed or loose footwear, elevating the foot as required and changing the dressing regularly by soaking.

Lateral avulsion and phenolization should be used for recurrent or chronic cases. A ring block is performed, the toe exanguinated and a tourniquet applied. Using Thwaite's nail nippers, a 3-mm strip is cut from the lateral edge of the nail (Figure 7.19a). The cut needs to be extended down to the germinal matrix under the nail fold. This may be achieved by retracting the proximal nail fold and extending the cut using a nail chisel (Figure 7.19b). The 3-mm strip is then avulsed using strong artery forceps, and granulation tissue is curetted from the fold. White soft paraffin is applied to the skin surrounding the cavity to protect it from phenol spills. A cotton bud is fashioned to an appropriate size, soaked in phenol (90%), pushed deep into the cavity and moved around to ensure penetration of the phenol into the deepest aspects of the germinal matrix. The phenol is applied for 3 minutes, and then the bud is removed. The cavity is gently irrigated with an alcoholic solution, such as hibitane, to deactivate excess phenol. The phenol usually achieves hemostasis, a dressing is applied and aftercare is as described above. If a nail is damaged and/or thickened, for example in onychogryphosis, then the nail may be completely avulsed and phenol applied to the entire germinal matrix to prevent regrowth.

(a)   (b)

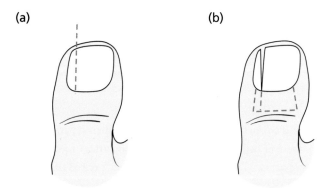

Figure 7.19 (a) A 3-mm strip is cut using Thwaite's nail nippers and (b) extended down to the germinal matrix under the nail fold.

Key points – surgical procedures

- Shave excision is an appropriate procedure for raised benign lesions; it can also be used to biopsy suspected basal cell carcinoma (BCC) or squamous cell carcinoma (SCC).
- Great care should be taken if punch biopsy is used on the nose, as it may result in a depressed and noticeable scar.
- Curettage is the most appropriate surgical intervention for seborrheic keratoses; curettage should be applied parallel to the skin surface to limit the insult to the dermis.
- The flap of redundant skin, known as a 'dog-ear', which sometimes arises during wound repair, should be excised; if left, it will heal, leaving a proud area.
- Cryosurgery is a painful procedure, which limits its use in children.
- It is good practice to supply patients with a written advice sheet after cryosurgery.
- Toenail surgery in primary care is best avoided in patients with diabetes, peripheral vascular disease and neuropathy.

Pathology

It is the responsibility of the surgeon to follow up pathology reports. Benign pathology reports usually need no action other than communication of the result to the patient (Table 8.1).

Surgical practice

Audit in minor surgery is advised. The surgeon should continually monitor complication and infection rates, provisional versus histological diagnosis, and the satisfaction of both the patient and the operator with the long-term cosmetic result. Meticulous record keeping is vital in surgery, as a complaint or litigation may ensue many years after the procedure. A minor surgery record that lists all the important aspects of the surgery performed should be stored either in the patient's personal medical record or as a collection within a loose-leaf folder (Figure 8.1). Written consent will depend on local requirements; however, any record should include a column to enable the recording of consent obtained.

Using this simple recording technique enables surgeons to examine many aspects of their surgical practice. Personal standards can be set for diagnosis and complication rates. When a surgeon falls outside the set standards, remedial measures can be taken to correct any deficiencies in the surgical set-up. These may include inadequate sterile techniques,

Key points – examining your practice

- Audit of minor surgical procedures should be performed regularly to ensure ongoing maintenance of standards and to promote improvement where appropriate.
- Meticulous record keeping is vital.
- Personal standards should be set for diagnosis and complication rates, and kept under review.
- The surgeon is responsible for following up pathology reports.

TABLE 8.1

Follow-up of pathology reports

Report	Action
Benign pathology	• Reassure the patient
Bowen's disease	
Incompletely excised	• Review the patient • Consider 5-fluorouracil cream, cryosurgery, curettage or further surgery • Warn the patient to minimize sun exposure
Fully excised	• Provide advice on early detection of skin cancer • Follow-up may be appropriate • Warn the patient to minimize sun exposure
Basal cell carcinoma (BCC)	
Incompletely excised	• Review for further surgery or onward referral
Fully excised	• Review wound for signs of recurrence in 3–4 months; if normal, reassure the patient • Warn the patient about signs of recurrence, which may occur as late as 5 years after surgery; the risk of a second primary BCC within 5 years is approximately 50% • Provide advice about sun exposure and early detection of skin cancer • Follow-up may be appropriate
Squamous cell carcinoma (SCC)	
Incompletely excised	• Review for further surgery or onward referral
Fully excised	• Review and advise as for 'BCC fully excised' • Remember the potential for metastasis, particularly for lesions on the lips or ears and in immunocompromised patients. If the margins are very close, consider formal re-excision of the scar with a 3–4-mm margin
Malignant melanoma	
Full or incomplete excision	• Refer to local expert urgently

inadequate lesion recognition or poor surgical skills. If one's practice falls well outside the expected standards, a surgeon should stop operating and undertake further supervised practice.

Minor surgery patient record sheet

Date of procedure	01/10/2007
Patient name	John Smith
Date of birth	02/12/1960
Provisional diagnosis	Lipoma, left forearm
Planned procedure	Excision of lipoma
Consent	Full written
Anesthetic and volume	2 mL lidocaine (2%) with epinephrine
Procedure taken	Lesion marked, anesthetized, skin incision 2 cm, lipoma identified and soft tissue dissection. Lipoma removed. Hemostasis difficult – some residual bleeding. Potential space closed with 4:0 Vycril × 2; skin closed with interrupted sutures 4:0 Ethilon × 4
Removal of sutures	7 days
Complications	At removal of sutures some bruising but healing well
Histology results	Lipoma

Figure 8.1 A file record for a patient undergoing excision of a lipoma.

Useful resources

UK

British Association of Dermatologists
4 Fitzroy Square
London W1T 5HQ
Tel: +44 (0)20 7383 0266
admin@bad.org.uk
www.bad.org.uk

British Dermatological Nursing Group
Gable House, 40 High Street
Rickmansworth, Herts WD3 1ER
Tel: +44 (0)1923 776568
admin@bdng.org.uk
www.bdng.org.uk

British Skin Foundation
4 Fitzroy Square
London W1T 5HQ
Tel: +44 (0)20 7391 6341
bsf@bad.org.uk
www.britishskinfoundation.org.uk

CancerBackup
3 Bath Place, Rivington Street
London EC2A 3JR
Tel: +44 (0)20 7696 9003
Helpline: 0808 800 1234
(Mon–Fri 9 AM–8 PM)
www.cancerbackup.org.uk

Cancer Research UK
PO Box 123, Lincoln's Inn Fields
London WC2A 3PX
Tel: +44 (0)20 7242 0200
www.cancerresearchuk.org

Primary Care Dermatology Society
Gable House, 40 High Street
Rickmansworth, Herts WD3 1ER
Tel: +44 (0)1923 711678
pcds@pcds.org.uk
www.pcds.org.uk

Skin Cancer Information Network
MARC'S (Melanoma and Related Skin Cancers) Line Resource Centre
c/o Wessex Cancer Trust
Bellis House, 11 Westwood Road
Southampton, Hants SO17 1DL
Tel: +44 (0)1722 415071
MARCSline@salisbury.nhs.uk
www.wessexcancer.org

Skin Care Campaign
www.skincarecampaign.org

Surgical Dressing Manufacturers Association
70 Egremont Road, Milnrow
Rochdale, Lancs OL16 4ES
www.sdma.org.uk

USA

American Academy of Dermatology
PO Box 4014, Schaumburg
IL 60618-4014
Tel: +1 847 240 1280
Toll-free: 1 866 503 7546
mrc@aad.org
www.aad.org

American Skin Association
346 Park Avenue South, 4th Floor
New York, NY 10010
Tel: +1 212 889 4858
Toll-free: 1 800 499 7546
info@americanskin.org
www.americanskin.org

The Skin Cancer Foundation
149 Madison Avenue, Suite 901
New York, NY 10016
Tel: +1 212 725 5176
Toll-free: 1 800 7546 490
info@skincancer.org
www.skincancer.org

International

DermNet NZ (New Zealand)
www.dermnetnz.org

Skin & Cancer Foundation Australia
Tel: +61 (0)2 8833 3000
www.skin.com.au

Further reading

Agnew KL, Gilchrest BA, Bunker CB. *Fast Facts: Skin Cancer.* Oxford: Health Press, 2005.

Ankrett V, Williams I. *Quick Reference Atlas of Dermatology.* Tunbridge Wells: MSL, 1999.

Bennett RG. *Fundamentals of Cutaneous Surgery.* St Louis: Mosby, 1988.

Bhutani LK. *Colour Atlas of Dermatology.* 5th edn. New Delhi: Mehta, 2006.

Brown JS. *Minor Surgery, A Text and Atlas.* 4th edn. London: Hodder Arnold, 2001.

Epstein E. *Skin Surgery.* 6th edn. Philadelphia: WB Saunders, 1987.

Jackson A, Colver G, Dawber R. *Cutaneous Cryosurgery, Principles and Clinical Practice.* 3rd edn. London: Informa Healthcare, 2005.

Lawrence C. *An Introduction to Dermatological Surgery.* 2nd edn. Oxford: Churchill Livingstone, 2002.

Leffell DJ, Brown MD. *Manual of Skin Surgery.* New York: Wiley-Liss, 1997.

Nimmo WS, Rowbotham DJ, Smith G. *Anaesthesia.* 2nd edn. Oxford: Blackwell Scientific, 1994.

Robinson JK, Arndt KA, LeBoit PE, Wintroub BU. *Atlas of Cutaneous Surgery.* Philadelphia: WB Saunders, 1996.

Roenigk R, Roenigk Jr HH. *Roenigk & Roenigk's Dermatologic Surgery, Principles and Practice.* 2nd edn. New York: Marcel Dekker, 1996.

Rounding C, Bloomfield S. Surgical treatments for ingrowing toenails. *Cochrane Database Syst Rev* 2003;1: CD001541. www.thecochranelibrary.com

Saleh M, Sodera VK. *Illustrated Handbook of Minor Surgery and Operative Technique*. London: Heinemann Medical, 1988.

Schofield J, Kneebone R. *Skin Lesions*. London: Chapman and Hall Medical, 1996.

Tetzlaff JE. *Clinical Pharmacology of Local Anaesthetics*. Boston: Butterworth Heinemann, 2000.

White G. *Color Atlas of Dermatology*. 3rd edn. London: Mosby, 2004.

Index

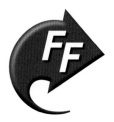

Fast Facts

the ultimate medical handbook series

- Concise, clear and practical

- Evidence-based and backed up with references

- The perfect balance of text, tables and illustrations

Other dermatology titles include:

Acne

Disorders of the Hair and Scalp

Eczema and Contact Dermatitis

Skin Cancer

Superficial Fungal Infections

New for 2008

Psoriasis, 3rd edn

Fast Facts are for practice, for reference, for teaching and for study.

For a full list visit:
www.fastfacts.com

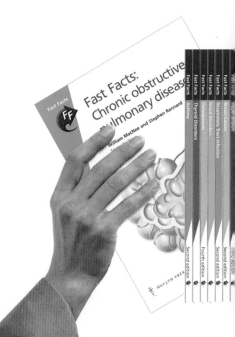

What the reviewers say:

www.fastfacts.com